TRACKING
A SHADOW

EDITH FORBES

TRACKING A SHADOW

My Lived Experiment with MS

GIRL FRIDAY BOOKS

GIRL FRIDAY BOOKS

Published by Girl Friday Books™, Seattle
www.girlfridaybooks.com

Cover design: Brad Foltz and Paul Barrett
Development & editorial: Devon Fredericksen
Production editorial: Dave Valencia

Image credits: cover © iStock Photo / ilbusca

ISBN (paperback): 978-1-954854-24-6
ISBN (e-book): 978-1-954854-25-3

Library of Congress Control Number: 2021918910

To Cherry and John, with love.

CONTENTS

PREFACE

FOLK DANCE WEEKEND
BECKET, MASSACHUSETTS

Like many people at the camp, the man ahead of me in the lunch line was at once familiar and a stranger. We had met in the whirl of the dance floor, briefly clasping hands to make circles and allemandes or wrapping arms around each other to swing, but we had not conversed. I knew only that he was a light-footed dancer with a bright smile.

Around us, the dining hall crowd was fizzing with happy energy, and when the stranger turned to speak to me, I anticipated a cheerful remark about the music or where we lived.

"I keep looking at you," he said, "because you look so much like a friend of mine who just died."

How does one respond to such an opening? The conventional "I'm sorry" might sound like "I'm sorry I look like your friend." Asking the obvious questions—Who was the friend? How did she die?—seemed intrusive.

Seeing that I was in a muddle, he quickly added, "It's good that you look like my friend. She was a lovely person, and I'm glad to be reminded of her. She was my doctor as well as a close friend."

"Was it . . . was she the same age we are?"

"She was fifty-four."

A few years younger than me.

"So it was untimely. Did she have cancer?" I asked. The automatic guess, for a female younger than sixty. Breast. Ovarian. Cervical.

"No, she had multiple sclerosis."

I flinched.

"That's a little spooky," I said. "Because I have multiple sclerosis."

Now he was the one at a loss, and I could almost see the thought balloon over his head: *I've just ruined her weekend.*

I smiled and assured him that I wasn't troubled by what he'd said. I was just startled by the coincidence.

He said, "I also had a great-aunt who had MS. She died of it when she was ninety-three."

We laughed. To anyone familiar with the wild variability of multiple sclerosis, this was an old joke.

At one extreme, the disease has cases like that reported in my local newspaper a few years ago, a college student diagnosed at age twenty and dead at age twenty-two. At the other extreme, it has the ninety-three-year-old great-aunt. In the middle, it has the fifty-four-year-old friend, a physician who presumably had up-to-date information and plenty of access to medical care before she died. The disease follows many pathways, and one can't know ahead of time which path it will take.

When my new acquaintance made the joke about his great-aunt, he was trying to banish the frightening specter he thought he had raised. In fact, he had not caused me any new anxiety. I had known for two decades that my disease could change from benign to devastating at any time.

What he had done was to reawaken an idea.

Some time before that dance weekend, I had been in a gap between projects, and my brother said, "Why don't you write about your experience with multiple sclerosis? I'll bet people would be interested."

I said, "I haven't had any experience. I'm perfectly healthy."

He said, "That's just the point."

But where was the story? Yes, the diagnosis had prompted me to make changes in my habits, but I did not know if my actions had made a difference. My good luck might be just that—luck. Many people with MS have minimal symptoms, regardless of what they do. My doctor could not say which it was, because my experimental strategy was my own and had never been the subject of a controlled study. I had no statistical data to put into a scholarly article, and I couldn't write a story about courageous struggle, because I hadn't yet needed any courage. So what was there to write about?

At some point, I realized that in my case the specifics of my strategy may have been less important than the simple fact that I *had* a strategy.

A diagnosis of multiple sclerosis is scary. One's mind immediately leaps to the worst-case images of incontinence, blindness, spasticity, and a future using a wheelchair. At the time of my first episode, the medical system had no answers. The disease would do whatever it was going to do, and its cause was unknown. The only advice was to live your life and hope that researchers would someday find a treatment.

But what exactly did it mean to "live your life" when life now included a permanent shadow companion that often sleeps but could cripple or kill when it wakes up?

1

A BUZZ IN
THE NERVES

In the fall of 1993, when I was thirty-eight years old, I noticed some peculiar neurological symptoms. On my left side, from my foot up my leg and torso to my thumb, my nerves prickled. Things my rational brain knew were cold, such as wet sneakers in a chilly rain, felt cold on my right foot but hot on my left.

My family doctor said the sensations might be nothing at all, a passing oddity, but if they were a symptom of a more serious condition, the three leading possibilities were a brain tumor, tertiary syphilis, or multiple sclerosis.

Listening to him, I wondered if he was always so forthright in presenting such sobering possibilities to his patients. He had known me a long time; perhaps he knew I liked a maximum of information and a minimum of medication. On my rare visits to the doctor, I always hoped he'd tell me that the remedy was time or a change in habits, not a drug or surgery. In most cases, he could oblige.

Dr. Hale had a booming bass voice and a joviality that sometimes felt overdone, as if he were covering some social uneasiness. Early in our acquaintance, his manner put me off a bit, and I did not fully appreciate his skill. When I knew him better, he served as a marvelously effective placebo, if placebo is defined as any remedy that works by harnessing the power of the mind.

I once strained a tendon or ligament in my thumb, and after two weeks the thumb was still painful, so I went to see Dr. Hale. He said I didn't need to do anything to fix the injury; it would get better on its own. I went home, and the next day the pain was gone.

This was typical of our doctor-patient relationship. He understood that what would fix me, as often as not, was information. Drugs were reserved for problems such as bacterial infections, when information was not enough.

In the case of my neurological symptoms, he laid out his analysis. The symptoms themselves were annoying but not debilitating, a pins-and-needles disturbance in my sensory nerves. Since I was in a monogamous relationship and had no other symptoms of venereal disease, tertiary syphilis was highly unlikely. If the neurological symptoms went away (which they soon did), that would rule out a brain tumor. To cover all bases, I had a test for Lyme disease, which came back negative. That left two possibilities: multiple sclerosis or the unexplained passing oddity.

In 1993 the medical treatment for both of these conditions was identical—nothing. Go live your life and see if the symptoms come back. Dr. Hale said I could have an

MRI and possibly learn if it was MS, but we agreed that it made more sense to wait for a recurrence.

At that time, I had only a casual knowledge of the disease. When I got home from the appointment, I pulled my big fat "complete medical guide" off the shelf and paged through to the letter *M*. It was a measure of either my good luck or a good constitution that in the midst of many well-thumbed books on nutrition, biology, natural history, and agriculture, the book about medical problems was crisp and shiny, almost untouched.

What I found is that the hallmark of MS is unpredictability. Some diseases, like the common cold, are a minor nuisance. Some diseases, like the lung cancer that killed my father, are a probable death sentence. Some diseases, like arthritis, are chronic and painful but can be managed and do not necessarily shorten life. Multiple sclerosis can be any of these things. Its symptoms can range from prickling in the nerves all the way to blindness, spasticity, incontinence, crippling fatigue, and premature death.

There are famous cases, like the cellist Jacqueline du Pré, whose career and then life were swiftly ended by the disease. There are the more ordinary cases, like a family friend who had occasional troubling flare-ups but generally lived a long and healthy life. Some people do well, others do badly, and medical science does not yet know why.

At the time of that first episode, I was impervious to worry because I was in a state of euphoria. A year earlier, the manuscript of my first novel had been plucked out of a publisher's slush pile, and a copy of the published book had just arrived in my mailbox. Far from fretting over dire possibilities in a medical text, I was busy ordering flowers to be delivered to my editor and others who worked at the press.

I lived on a beautiful small farm in Vermont. My days were divided between physical work outdoors and hours at my desk working on another novel. In summer I played on a softball team and planted a garden. In winter I cross-country skied. Life was good, and I was not in a mood to be concerned about a hypothetical problem. The symptoms were gone, and there was nothing to be done anyway.

Eighteen months later, in the spring of 1995, the symptoms came back. The prickling now extended to my other foot and my whole hand, and I also experienced Lhermitte's sign, an electric zing that traveled down my spine when I bent my head forward. This time Dr. Hale recommended that I see a neurologist. He referred me to a staff physician at a nearby medical center.

The neurologist, Dr. Sage, was a lean, scholarly looking man with an air of dignified reserve and a quiet, pleasant voice. He reminded me of the family doctor from my childhood, who was likewise tall, gaunt, and dignified, with a deep, soothing voice that made me want him to keep talking. Even as I was squirming in dread at being stabbed with a needle, I had seen him as wise and kind.

In the Wyoming ranching community where I grew up, doctors in general were notable people, but this doctor made a particular impression because he was so unlike most of our neighbors. As a child I just thought, *His accent is different, his manner is different, and everyone seems to think he's really smart.* Not until I was older did I realize that he was Jewish.

In the early drafts of my first novel, which was set in that part of the country, I had used this doctor as a character in the story. Of all the characters in the manuscript, he was the only one who was based directly on a real person. Then an urban friend of mine, who is Jewish, read the manuscript and squawked, "I can't believe you used such a stereotype character, the small-town doctor who is really smart and the only Jew in the town."

It didn't matter that our real doctor was exactly that. His family was the only Jewish family in the town. His kids were high achievers, smart, musical, and artistic. He was real, but in fiction he became a stereotype. In the next draft of my book, I rewrote the doctor character to be some unspecified ethnicity and took away an important lesson about writing fiction: don't ever try to use a real person as a character.

At the time of my referral to Dr. Sage, I was forty years old and had had only two medical interventions of any consequence at all. The first was when I was six years old and dislocated my elbow falling off a horse.

It was March, calving season on my family's ranch, and I had gone along with some of my family and the ranch crew to round up the pregnant cows from a large pasture and bring them closer to the barns before they calved. As the cattle approached the barns, my horse lagged behind the other horses. When he broke into a gallop to catch up, I lost my stirrups and landed on the ground.

Initially, I didn't realize I was hurt. I was too angry and embarrassed at having fallen off my horse. I kept insisting that the only reason I fell off was that my stupid little snow boots had made my feet come out of the stirrups. I didn't consider it an excuse that I was six years old and the horse was a big, rough-gaited, jugheaded, hardmouthed lunk with an evil eye and ugly pink skin under his white coat, a horse named Higgins that no one else liked but I, for some unknown reason, had been begging to ride. My mother had finally given in and permitted me to ride him, probably because, as a single woman with seven children and a cattle ranch to run, she had no energy left to argue with me.

After the mishap, I was too busy complaining about my snow boots to notice my elbow, and no one else did either. One of my sisters drove me back to our house, where I could rest and get warm, while everyone else went on with the cattle work, which had to get done. Eventually, another sister found me in the bathroom crying because I needed to pee and couldn't bend my elbow to push my pants down. She helped me with the pants and then drove me into town to the hospital.

For anesthesia, the doctor put a cotton mask over my face and dripped ether onto it long enough to pop my elbow back into place. I woke up in a hospital bed with my arm in a sling and my mother's get-well gift of a beautiful edition of *Winnie the Pooh*, which cheered me up considerably.

The second intervention was the extraction of my wisdom teeth when I was in my twenties. Anesthesia had evolved beyond an ether drip, but the procedure was similarly uneventful. Other than that, I'd had a couple of rounds of antibiotics, for possible strep throat and a poison ivy reaction that became infected, and I'd had occasional checkups and vaccinations.

Basically, I was very lucky. My health was good, and I had an ongoing relationship with a local family doctor. My medical bills were minimal, and I'd always paid them myself. I did have insurance but had never come close to meeting its high deductible. My referral to Dr. Sage would be my first personal encounter with the wider health-care system.

At my first consultation with Dr. Sage, I described my symptoms, and he did a physical examination that included neurological tests. At one point, he attached electrodes to determine whether the abnormality was in the peripheral nerves of my arms and legs or in the central nervous system, in my brain and spine. The test showed that the problem was in the central nervous system, which was consistent with multiple sclerosis but not conclusive.

Dr. Sage recommended that I have further testing. He took out a pad and began to write down the tests he recommended. An MRI of the brain. An MRI of the spine. A spinal tap. Various blood tests.

"How much does each of these cost?" I asked. "I have a high deductible, and I'll be paying for them myself."

He paused and looked down at his list.

"Perhaps we could start with some of the tests and see what they show. Then we can decide about the others."

He was gracious and matter of fact. We discussed the various costs. In 1995, MRIs were about $1,500 each. The spinal tap around $800. The blood work a few hundred. I said if the tests were vital, I could pay for them, but I only wanted to do what was really necessary. We agreed that I would have the blood tests, the brain MRI, and the spinal tap. We would wait and see about the spine MRI.

As he wrote down the orders, I pondered how his thinking had changed when he learned the cost would be paid by me and not by the distant and seemingly bottomless resources of an insurance company. Instead of being governed by what the insurance company would or would not reimburse, the doctor and I had to make our own cost-benefit analysis and decide what was needed.

The next question to arise was scheduling. Dr. Sage said the spinal tap could be done quite soon, because he would do it himself in his own office. Whenever the medical professionals talked about this procedure, they called it a "lumbar puncture," but I tried to stick with "spinal tap." To my ear, "puncture" conjured up images of flat tires and rusty-nail wounds that lead to tetanus, while "tap" suggested foaming mugs of beer and maple trees during the spring sap run.

When the time came, I lay on my side, curled forward to spread the vertebrae apart, and he inserted the needle into my lower back to draw off a sample of fluid. The procedure gave me the same weird, uneasy sensation as dental drilling under novocaine. Any pain was negligible, but for a couple of days afterward I felt a reluctance to touch or move the site of needle insertion, the breach in the central nervous system.

Unlike the spinal tap, the MRI was done in a separate department and involved the larger hospital schedule. Since my situation was not immediately life threatening, I had to wait for several weeks. By the time of the MRI, my symptoms had gone away, except for a small patch of numbness on my left thumb.

Multiple sclerosis typically begins as a relapsing/remitting disease. The relapses, or flare-ups, last a few weeks. The length of remission varies widely, from months to years. During a relapse, there are lesions of active inflammation of the myelin in the central nervous system. When the relapse ends, some sites of inflammation may heal, while others leave scarring behind. ("Sclerosis" means "scarring.") If I did have MS, the delay in getting the MRI meant that I was now in remission and only the lesions that had left scarring would show up on the image.

Apart from the awareness that the result might be some dreadful diagnosis, having an MRI was a bit like a futuristic theme park experience, the closest I was likely to come to feeling like a space traveler. Everything in the room with the machine was clean, shiny, and plastic. A technician sat at a console behind a panel of glass. Sliding into the tube, I could imagine I was being inserted into a pod for cryopreservation.

The challenge was staying still for half an hour. Being told to keep perfectly still made every nerve and muscle in my body want to move. Fortunately, the machine made an entertaining array of noises, rather like a crew of construction workers in some distant part of the house. First a rapid-fire jackhammer. Then a nail gun, methodically working its way along a floorboard. Then quieter pulses of tapping, someone knocking on drywall looking for the stud, followed by some intermittent deep thumps, armloads of lumber dumped on the floor. Then back to the jackhammer, a smaller one this time.

The time passed reasonably quickly, and a technician came to slide me out of the tube. I retrieved my watch and glasses and went home to await the results. As a diagnostic procedure, the MRI was nonintrusive, almost restful. It beat the heck out of the breast-flattening pinch plates of a mammogram back then.

At my follow-up appointment, Dr. Sage said the results of the tests were inconclusive. The brain scan showed no lesions. The spinal tap and blood tests showed slight indications consistent with MS but not definitively. The blood tests had ruled out alternatives, such as Lyme disease, and my symptoms were typical of early MS, but he could not confirm a diagnosis.

I asked, "Suppose it is in fact MS. Is there anything I should do to improve the outlook?"

He said the same thing Dr. Hale had said. "No, not really; just live your life." During relapses, patients often received steroids to try to reduce the damage from inflammation, but there weren't yet any medications aimed at preventing relapses.

I asked about diet, exercise, stress, and lifestyle in general.

He said it was undoubtedly helpful to stay fit, eat a healthy diet, and not subject myself to unnecessary stress, but there weren't any specific things to do or avoid. Then he added, "If you have an interest in alternative medicine, some practitioners recommend evening primrose oil, but there isn't any scientific data on the topic."

My immediate reaction was frustration at the uncertainty. In the time I was waiting for test results, I had read more about the disease, and I thought it was very likely what I had. So why couldn't he say so?

2

EXPERIMENT IN
THE LIVING ROOM

Although both doctors had said there was nothing to be done, I was not content with this answer. I needed to do something. If nothing else, I could study meditation in order to be at peace with helplessness.

I was raised by a mother who viewed any barricade in her path as something to be overcome, whether by leaping over it, by bulldozing it flat, or, most commonly, by locating the person who knew where there was a gate. She could be stoic, but she was never passive.

Both of my parents came from old Boston families. They grew up in a world where private schools, travel, and household staff were the norm, but the women wore sensible shoes, and the only purpose of shopping was to replace objects that had worn out. They took vacation trips to Europe and returned to houses where the faded wallpaper was left as it was, not because there was no money to replace it, but because the paper still had a few more years or decades of use left in it. In the 1800s, their family's wealth was new, the product of entrepreneurship. By the 1900s, it had become a savings account, a resource to be conserved and passed along to children.

In the 1930s, my father became interested in ranching and began spending more and more of his time in Wyoming. In 1939, my mother dropped out of Vassar College to marry him. Together, they left New England behind and settled in Wyoming for good.

My father had attended Harvard in the era when admission was based on pedigree more than merit. On his ranch, he embarked on an experiment in the opposite direction. He wanted to evaluate cattle based on their practical merit rather than their pedigree. He hoped to develop a working model of scientific selection methods that would revolutionize cattle breeding.

In that era (the 1940s and 1950s), there were two separate worlds in livestock production. The commercial growers raised meat for people to eat. The purebred breeders raised pedigree animals and competed with one another to win prizes in the show ring. The criteria in show judging were as arbitrary as the fashions in clothing and had little to do with the practical needs of growing food. In some cases, the show ring fads led to the propagation of serious genetic defects.

My father wanted to unite the two worlds. He thought pedigree cattle should be selected to improve traits that were useful in food production. He wanted to measure those useful traits and analyze the data. Today this seems like an obvious thing to do, but in 1950, it was a radical idea and was not well received in many quarters of a very conservative industry.

The petri dish for his experiment was a new breed of cattle called Red Angus. The Black Angus breed carried an occasional recessive gene for a red coat, but the Black Angus breed association would not register its red calves. My father and a few like-minded breeders began to collect the rejected red calves to use as the foundation for a new breed on which they could test their ideas. In addition to the usual requirements of pedigree and breed type, the Red Angus registry would include the novel requirement that the breeder measure each animal's growth rate so that cattle could be selected to improve this important practical trait.

Eight years into his experiment and a year before I was born, my father was diagnosed with lung cancer.

Over the next two years, the family shuttled back and forth between Wyoming and Massachusetts, as my father was in and out of the hospital. When we were in Boston for his surgeries, the youngest of us stayed at my grandmother's house while the older ones were scattered among other relatives. My mother more or less camped at the hospital. In the course of his treatment, my father became the subject of what was then a new and experimental procedure, a surgery to remove part of his second lung after one entire lung had already been removed.

When my father died, some of my mother's relatives urged her to sell the ranch in Wyoming and bring her children permanently back to Boston, where she would have the support of a large extended family. My mother did not follow their advice. She loved Wyoming and thought it was a good place for kids to grow up. She wanted to carry on the dream my father was pursuing when he died.

Her situation as a single mother whose seven children ranged in age from fourteen years down to fourteen months didn't stop her. Nor did the conservative, male-dominated culture of the 1950s beef industry, which did not welcome a woman with bright ideas. She simply didn't accept other people telling her what was possible.

When I was about seven years old, a woman who briefly worked in our household described my mother as a tornado. I instantly hated the woman and was ready to scratch her eyes out.

Years later, I might have used the same word myself.

My mother needed to be a tornado. Along with the idealistic dream of bringing innovation to agriculture, my father's death had left her with the daily reality of seven children, several hundred head of cattle, a crew of employees and their families, and a large expanse of land that, in addition to grass, yucca, and wildlife, held an array of barns, fences, machinery, and irrigation ditches, all needing maintenance. Throughout my childhood, she had too much to do and far too little time. Just the family and the business made for a full load, never mind changing the world.

She was the opposite of a Patient Griselda. She did not quietly accept what life brought her, because life had brought too many bad things. A mother hospitalized for depression. A sister dead in childbirth. Another sister who killed herself. And above all my father's cancer. If my mother ever uttered the serenity prayer, it was only after she had investigated every possible avenue of resistance first.

Being a bookish introvert, I found her energy exhausting and sometimes embarrassing. Of all the parents in our rural neighborhood, she was the only one who showed up dressed in a costume for the Halloween party at our two-room elementary school. And it wasn't a "regular" costume with a commercial witch's mask or a princess tiara. It was a bizarre homemade concoction consisting of a mop for a wig, a red bandanna masking her face, a voluminous green poncho covering her body from head to foot, and my great-grandfather's Union Army cavalry sword in her hand. Fortunately, the year was 1966, and everyone in the neighborhood knew her, so nobody called the police.

The thing about parents, though, is that we *are* them, whether we like it or not. My mother was adventurous, impatient, energetic, tenacious, and skeptical of authority. I can be all of those things too. Every attribute in her that bugged me is also part of me.

Another part of me is the product of a ghost. I was only a year old when my father died, but he was a presence in our household throughout my childhood, as our ranch continued the experiment he had launched.

In farming generally, there is no separation between livelihood and daily life. One lives in the workplace, and one's schedule is governed by the weather and the tasks at hand. In our case, the ranch and the cattle became a laboratory, and our house was the place where the information from my father's experiment was recorded and analyzed.

Computers were far in the future. Measurements were tabulated with pens and rulers on legal-sized pads of paper, and stacks of my mother's "papers" were scattered all over our house. She kept a portable office table in the living room so she could work there while my brother and I played with plastic farm animals and toy trucks on the rug.

The moment we were old enough to do math, we were recruited to help with the papers. We learned the vocabulary of what was known as "performance testing" and terms like "adjusted weaning weight" and "cow efficiency." We learned the formulas to convert raw data into standardized measurements for comparison. We typed up tables of data to supply to the people buying our cattle. And, although we knew our ranch was considered a maverick by the traditional beef industry, we shared our mother's belief that we were the ones headed in the right direction.

Over the next few decades, because of my mother and other forward-thinking people, the ideas that were considered crackpot in 1955 would spread through the industry, grow steadily more sophisticated, and become well established. By the time I was facing a medical decision in the 1990s, I'd had a lifetime of training in the value of good data.

In a sense, I did not have to make a medical decision, because Dr. Sage had not said, definitively, that I had MS. Instead, what he told me and also wrote in my record was that I had some symptoms possibly indicative of early MS, but the brain MRI was negative, and I had no confirmed diagnosis.

His notes in my record did not point out that I had not had an MRI of my spine, nor did he encourage me to get one. And yet something in our conversation, perhaps the mention of evening primrose oil, made me think that his unspoken opinion was actually similar to mine. It was quite likely that I had MS.

Only later did it occur to me that he might have hedged for a nonmedical reason: insurance.

Given the practical realities of the insurance system at that time, I would not be helped by a diagnosis of MS. If I did have it, I was in remission, and there were no medications to prescribe. Since there were no medications, I did not need a diagnosis to get my insurance company to pay for treatment.

On the other hand, if he did put a positive diagnosis of MS into my medical record, I would forever be a prisoner of my insurance coverage, because no other carrier would ever insure me at anything like my current premiums, if they agreed to insure me at all.

This was a predicament familiar to me from personal experience. Not because I had been in it myself. Because someone else had been, and I had been the beneficiary of that person's misfortune.

My first serious job after college was working for a software company with about eighty employees. After I was hired, I found out that I had not been the company's first choice for the job. They had wanted to hire another applicant, but she was getting treatment for Hodgkin's disease, and the company's health insurance carrier refused to add her to the company policy.

So the other candidate was forced to stay at her old job in order to keep her health insurance, and the software company was forced to hire the person they thought was the lesser candidate—me.

Regardless of the vagaries of our insurance system and what Dr. Sage had written in my medical record, my gut was telling me I probably did have MS, and I should plan accordingly. Faced with a disease that could become crippling, I was incapable of doing nothing. I needed to take action, and, like a homing pigeon headed for its familiar place, I headed to a library to see what I could learn about the disease.

3

SHELVES OF BAFFLEMENT

For most of my family, books had been a childhood defense against boredom and frustration. My mother was so over-whelmingly busy that we often found ourselves sitting in a car or at some appointed meeting place waiting for her to finish with her errands, and we learned never to go anywhere without taking a book.

On one occasion that became part of family legend, my next-older sister was due to fly home from college, and everyone forgot about her flight. When someone finally remembered, a long time later, we piled into the car and raced to the county airport, bursting with apologies. Instead of being met with tears and reproaches, we found my sister placidly settled on an airport bench reading her book. It had not even crossed her mind to find change for the pay phone and call to say she was there. She was accustomed to my mother being late for almost everything and assumed that her ride would arrive eventually.

In my current dilemma, the library of choice was the one at the medical center where I had seen Dr. Sage. It had an excellent reading room for the general public, and when I scanned the shelves of books, I saw that the section on multiple sclerosis was one of the larger sections. At first I thought, *Great! There's lots of information.* As I started reading, I discovered that the quantity of material was a measure of bafflement, not knowledge.

With most common diseases, doctors have at least some solid information to impart to their patients. They may have a vaccine to prevent it, or a medication to cure it, or a treatment that at least slows its progress. They may be able to explain factors that increase risk, like smoking, or sun exposure, or overeating. Or if they don't know the cause or the risk factors and they don't have a treatment, they may at least be able to describe in detail what effects the disease will have.

With multiple sclerosis, the doctors could not say anything very definite about any of those things. They did not know what caused it; they did not know what factors might heighten risk; and they had no prevention measures, no cure, and only very limited symptomatic treatments. They could not even say with any certainty how the disease would manifest in a particular patient. In the early stage, the symptoms seemed to appear out of nowhere, grip the patient for some unpredictable period of time, and then disappear into the mist. Later, they might start to linger. Or the disease might attack a different function. No one knew what triggered the attacks or why they went away.

What scientists did understand was the "how," the basic mechanism of the disease. It is an autoimmune disease, meaning that the immune system attacks the body's own tissue as if it were a pathogen. There are many different autoimmune diseases, each defined by the particular type of tissue that is affected. In the case of MS, the targeted tissue is myelin, a fatty coating that protects and insulates nerve fibers. During an MS flare-up, the cells of the immune system start attacking the protective myelin in the central nervous system, like microscopic mice chewing through the plastic insulation on the electric wires in a house.

With the insulation gone, the wires develop static and short circuits. Nerve signals don't transmit properly. Depending on where and how much insulation is lost, the resulting symptoms can be anything from mild numbness and tingling to vision loss, spasticity, loss of balance, loss of bladder control, and cognitive impairment. For many people, the attacks are accompanied by debilitating fatigue.

Early in the course of the disease, the attacks usually end as abruptly as they start. The body repairs the damaged myelin, and the symptoms diminish or disappear. Before the MRI was developed, this relapsing/remitting pattern of symptoms had been a key marker for diagnosing MS.

Other peculiarities had aided diagnosis. One was Lhermitte's sign, the electric sensation down the spine that I had experienced. Another was that symptoms became more pronounced if body temperature was raised. In pursuit of diagnosis, patients had sometimes been placed in a very hot bath. If the symptoms intensified, the diagnosis became more certain. Even before the advent of MRI, the hot bath method was generally abandoned, because doctors decided it might not be wise to subject patients to a process that made their symptoms worse.

By 1995, MRI had become the standard diagnostic tool for MS, and most researchers were working at the molecular level to study the immune system and the mechanism of the disease. In previous decades, though, the research had largely operated at the macro level of history and epidemiology. When was the disease first identified? Where was it prevalent? What were the characteristics of populations with a high incidence of the disease?

Because the disease was so mysterious, researchers had delved into these questions with a passion, looking for anything that might be a clue to the cause or a treatment. Now I pored over their findings, hoping to notice something they had missed. Reading through that shelf of bafflement and speculation was like reading a whodunit in which the culprit had not yet been identified.

Historically, multiple sclerosis was considered a "new" disease, in the sense that there was a moment in time when it first began to be observed in autopsies. The disease leaves a distinct pattern of damage in the central nervous system, a pattern that had not been reported prior to the 1800s. In the mid-1800s, a handful of reports appeared. As decades passed, the reports became more and more numerous. Now, in the United States, it is estimated that about half a million people have MS.

Had something happened in the 1800s that could explain the appearance of this new disease? The obvious new development in the 1800s and beyond was the

Industrial Revolution and its attendant urbanization. Could some social, environmental, or technological change that came with industrialization be a factor in MS?

The books had long sections describing the epidemiology of the disease, as researchers looked for possible risk factors. Some populations had a very high incidence of MS; other populations had almost none.

The disease was rare in people who grew up in the tropics. It was prevalent in people who grew up farther from the equator, where the climate was temperate. However, it wasn't prevalent in all places with cooler climates. There were large exceptions. The disease was rare in China and Japan. It was rare among Inuits. Even in places where it was common, such as Scandinavia, it was more common inland than it was near the coast.

There was an instance when the disease had suddenly become prevalent, on the Faroe Islands, off the coast of Denmark. The disease was unknown there until after World War II, when a large contingent of British soldiers was stationed on the island. Had the soldiers brought a virus with them? Or something else? No one had been able to isolate an MS virus, on the Faroe Islands or anywhere else.

My entire life had been shaped by ranching and farming, so when I studied the map of MS distribution, I thought about agriculture. I also liked to cook, so I thought about cuisines. What leapt out when I looked through those two lenses was a distinct agricultural and culinary difference in the areas with high incidence. To find out if this impression was supported by more specific data, I visited the library at a nearby agricultural college.

In a textbook, I found what I was looking for: a map of the distribution of dairy cattle. It was an almost one-to-one mapping onto the distribution of MS. The major exception was India, which had significant milk production but low MS incidence. But in the temperate climates, all countries with high MS incidence had high milk production, and all countries where MS was rare had little or no milk production.

Later I would mention this observation to my brother-in-law John, who is a research physician studying immunological approaches to cancer. He promptly did a search of medical journals and sent me an article from a recent study in France. In specific numbers and statistical analysis, the article reported the same correlation I had noticed: with the exception of a few areas in the tropics, MS incidence paralleled milk consumption.

If milk did turn out to be a risk factor, there could be various explanations for the exceptions in the tropics. Perhaps climate was also a factor. Perhaps the risk element in milk depended on the conditions under which the cattle were raised. However, as I often reminded myself, it was also possible that the correlation in temperate climates was a coincidence, and there was no causal connection between milk and MS.

For myself personally, a connection to milk would be gloomy news. I was a lifelong dairy queen, passionately fond of all things milk. I slathered my bread with butter. I poured lavish cream into my coffee and tea. My usual snack was sharp cheddar melted on crackers. I loved cream sauces, creamy desserts, ice cream, sour cream, clotted cream on scones, and crème caramel. I put cheese on anything Mexican or Italian and cooked in butter at every opportunity.

When I was a child, our ranch had its own Ayrshire and Guernsey milk cows and its own cream separator. The separator spun the milk so that the lighter part, the cream, went out one spout, while the heavier skimmed milk went out another. The separator could be set to produce different levels of butterfat in the cream, and occasionally ours would get set to a level where the cream was so thick it had to be spooned. When that happened, I was in paradise. I would spoon cream onto my Rice Krispies and stir the whole bowl into a single lump of luscious, creamy crunchiness.

I really didn't like the idea that MS might be related to milk. On the other hand, if there *was* a link, I wanted to know about it.

As I went on reading, my antennae were alert for anything connected to diet and especially milk. Because no drugs were available at that time, the books about living with MS had a lot of theories about lifestyle, especially diet. The most common recommendation was to eat a low-fat diet. Another recommendation, only partly contradictory, was to take supplements of evening primrose oil.

Evening primrose oil is a concentrated source of a fatty acid called gamma linolenic acid (GLA), which is a component of myelin. The idea behind taking it as a supplement was that it might help the body rebuild damaged myelin or compensate for a deficiency.

Pursuing this line of reasoning, researchers in England had done a study to see if MS patients would benefit from eating margarine made from sunflower oil, which was also a good source of GLA. (Sunflower oil was not as rich in GLA as evening primrose oil, but it was much less expensive.) The study concluded that the patients who used sunflower oil margarine did do somewhat better than the controls who had not changed their diet.

Reading the result of the sunflower oil study, I could see several possible explanations. The direct explanation was that GLA was indeed helpful. The indirect explanation was that the patients eating sunflower margarine were not eating butter, so it was the elimination of butter that was beneficial. The complex explanation was that both adding GLA and eliminating butter were helpful.

Another line of thought in the MS literature was that the oils in fish might be beneficial. This was partly based on the observation that in Scandinavia, people who lived on the coast had a lower incidence of MS than people who lived inland.

Like the margarine study, and in fact like many theories about diet and disease, an observed connection to a particular food can have either a positive or negative interpretation. Did the benefit come from eating more fish or from eating less of what the inland population was eating instead of fish? Is the Mediterranean diet healthy because of the presence of olive oil or because of the absence of Coke and potato chips?

It made sense to me that diet might change the composition of a body component like myelin. My family's business was in livestock production, where feed rations were systematically designed to produce desirable qualities in the meat, eggs, or milk of the animals being fed.

When I was growing up, before people started worrying about their arteries, the desirable fat in animal products was the type that came from feeding the animals a lot of corn. The corn-fed fat was harder at room temperature because it had more saturated fat and less of the fats now considered desirable, the healthy omega-3 polyunsaturated fats. (Besides being harder, the corn-fed fat also tasted really good.) Nowadays, the trend is to grow beef cattle entirely on grass to increase the level of omega-3 fats in their meat and to feed crops like flaxseed to chickens and pigs for the same purpose.

If the body composition of other mammals could be altered by their diet, presumably ours could too. I didn't know if myelin could be changed in the way that superficial body fat could be changed, but the idea was cause for curiosity.

Eventually, I reached the end of the shelf of MS books and also a saturation point in my own brain. The sum total of the recommendations in the books was similar to what Dr. Sage had said. Living a healthy lifestyle and avoiding stress couldn't hurt, but there were no specific recommendations with any weight of medical research behind them.

It was not that dietary strategies had been comprehensively researched and shown to be irrelevant. There just wasn't much research data on the effect of diet. Some of the questions that intrigued me, particularly about milk, had never been studied at all. So I was left to decide for myself if I wanted to "do" anything or simply live my life exactly as I always had.

In all of the previous instances that my family doctor had told me I didn't need to do anything, the message had meant something very different from what it meant now. In those past instances, such as my sprained thumb, he was telling me the problem would get better on its own, so I could leave it alone.

That was not the message now. The message now was that the problem would do whatever it was going to do, and I just had to wait and see how bad it would get.

At the time I was making the decision, I did not think about my parents or my own history. I just did what I felt driven to do. But looking back, I realize that my strategy was rooted in my history.

Thanks to my mother, I wasn't good at waiting to see what happened, especially if the something might be really, really bad. I needed to take action.

Thanks to my father, the action that felt logical and natural was to embark on an experiment. In this case, the lab rat would be me.

Based on what I had learned about the disease, I decided to make three specific changes in my habits. I would stop eating any milk products whatsoever. I would start eating more vegetable oil. And I would start taking a basic multivitamin and a calcium supplement to make up for nutrients I would lose without the milk.

I didn't know if these changes would help, but they were consistent with the most important principle in medicine. They could do no harm.

4

COROLLARY
BENEFITS

I did not like giving up milk. For one thing, I was very fond of it. But beyond that, I had always been irritated by people who grilled waiters about the ingredients in every item on the menu or snooped through the dishes on the potluck table in search of toxins or political incorrectness.

Now I had become one of those people. I had a "dietary restriction," and what was worse, I didn't even have a doctor's order to justify it. It was my own idea.

When I could, I kept my mouth shut and ate the things I could see had no milk, like fruit salad and roast beef and plain rice. I loved Asian restaurants because I could eat anything on the menu. Italian restaurants were a challenge, but I found that restaurant people were very nice about requests for "no cheese," and my dinner companions never had any desire to snitch a slice of my pizza.

For home cooking, our farm and garden had been pro-
ducing chicken, beef, eggs, vegetables, and berries for many
years, and we continued to rely on them. At other people's
houses, though, it didn't work to stay quiet and eat what
I could. My hosts would notice and ask, and soon most
friends were adjusting their dinner menus on my behalf.

In one way I was very fortunate. At about the same
time I adopted a dietary quirk, lots of other people did too.
Soy milk suddenly escaped its little niche beside the echi-
nacea and brewer's yeast in health-food stores and began
appearing in ordinary supermarkets. Within a few years,
I could find several brands of soy milk at the Safeway in
my Wyoming hometown, and any notion of originality was
dispelled. I was part of a fad.

Multiple sclerosis operates on a long time schedule, and I
expected it might take years to know if my diet was helping. However, with other aspects of my health, I noticed
changes very quickly.

The first change was that I lost a lot of weight. For
years I had fluctuated between 132 and 136 pounds, a
normal weight for five foot seven. Within a few months,
I had dropped to 122 pounds, even though I was eating
like a horse. Avoiding milk products, especially cheese, had
eliminated a lot of fat calories. Also, since almost any dessert worth eating contains butter, cream, milk, or all three,
I was eating very few desserts.

In the United States, a person won't make herself popu-
lar complaining that she's getting too thin and needs to eat
more, but that was the case with me. I began to experiment

with recipes and figured out substitutions that would let me make desserts and rich sauces again. In piecrust, I replaced butter with lard. In cakes and beef stroganoff, I replaced sour cream with a mixture of mayonnaise and soy milk. I used almond butter to make cookies and to spread on toast. In place of melted butter, I put vegetable oil on cooked vegetables. Gradually, as I worked more fat into my diet, my weight came back up and stabilized, a few pounds lighter than it had been, but okay for my height.

Along with my weight, my cholesterol also dropped. Prior to the diet changes, it had been squarely normal. At my first routine physical after the change, it had dropped twenty-five points to the lower end of normal.

One pleasant change was my hay fever. As a farmer, I spent every summer putting up hay, and my seasonal allergy to ragweed had been getting worse and worse. It had reached a point where I spent much of August and September dripping, sneezing, feverish, and dopey, wishing I could detach my head from my neck and store it on a shelf somewhere. Antihistamines helped, but they had side effects I didn't like, and I took as few as I could.

After a few months on my new food regimen, I discovered that my hay fever had diminished. If I put my face into a ragweed plant, I still would sneeze, but I no longer spent a month or two in a global state of allergic misery.

Over time, I also noticed a change in my experience with poison ivy. I'd had some very violent reactions in the past, and sometimes the reaction had seemed to take on a life of its own, spreading to places far from direct exposure, such as my abdomen. At the sites of direct exposure, the initial pinhead bubbles had inflamed into large, angry eruptions that looked like cheese under the broiler, swollen blisters weeping yellowish ooze. On one occasion, the blisters became infected and needed antibiotics.

In the years after changing my eating habits, I had no severe reactions. Direct contact with poison ivy still caused the localized pinhead blisters, but I never again had a reaction where the eruptions grew and spread into an angry, oozing mess.

I couldn't be sure these changes were related to my diet. Possibly I had washed more carefully. Possibly I had simply aged out of the allergies. My observations were an uncontrolled experiment, with a sample size of one. From a scientific point of view, the data was meaningless. For myself, however, I didn't care if the result was chance or an example of the placebo effect. As long as the result was good, I would keep following the strategy.

As much as physical benefit, my reduced allergies brought social and psychological benefits. For one thing, I now had an answer when someone asked why I avoided milk.

In those early years, I was reluctant to talk to casual acquaintances about the possibility that I had MS, never mind its possible connection to milk, for a whole sequence of reasons. First, I did not know for sure that I had MS, and I did not want to make a tempest in a teapot about my health. Second, even if I did have the disease, I did not know for sure that it was connected to milk. Third, even if the disease did have a connection to milk, I didn't know if it helped to change habits after the disease had already started. It felt like tying very slender threads with very weak knots to compose an explanation in which every sentence began, "There's a chance that . . ."

At that time, my "symptoms" consisted of a small patch of numbness on one thumb. I was almost conspicuously healthy, throwing hay bales all summer and skiing in the Canadian Ski Marathon in the winter. It was possible I had simply invented all the patterns I was seeing.

When I found that my hay fever had improved, I latched on to the change as a social life raft. If anyone asked about the milk issue, I could say, "Staying away from milk seems to help my respiratory allergies." The explanation was true, as far as it went, and occasionally the questioner reported having observed the same thing or had heard of someone else who had.

Even more than social ease, the improvement in my allergies provided a Pavlovian reward that reinforced my decision to change my habits. I thought, *Here is a bit of evidence that milk has an effect on my immune system. It's one little piece of data suggesting I might not be nuts.* Regardless of what happened with MS, I was getting a concrete benefit from my diet, here and now.

I'm not sure I could have stuck with my decision if there had been no perceptible benefit to my health. A lack of deterioration doesn't register as a "benefit," emotionally. MS is a chancy disease, and I couldn't know what would have happened if I had done nothing.

The multiplicity of my own doubts, the daily need to go without foods I liked, and the constant awareness that I was causing a nuisance for other people might well have combined to wear down my resolve. As it was, physiology or chance had handed me a pellet of reward, and I kept going.

• • •

Many things happened in the next few years, mostly unrelated to my health. The summer after my flare-up, my partner's brother, a low-key, witty gay man who worked as a lawyer for Catholic Charities, died of leukemia, the same disease that had killed his father. My family's ranch in Wyoming, which contends with the same up and down cycles as all agricultural businesses, was thriving. Two more of my books were published.

Then, in fairly close succession, I sold my farm machinery and leased out my land in Vermont, built a new house on a corner of the farm, and ended my long-term relationship, in all cases with painful regret but also relief. A year or so after this series of upheavals, I began dating the woman I would marry.

More globally, my home state of Vermont passed the nation's first civil union law. Bill Clinton survived impeachment, and the younger Bush succeeded him as president. The US economy left behind the dot-com bubble and embarked on the housing bubble. The September 11 attacks and America's reaction to them knocked the world off one track and onto another, destination unknown.

Throughout most of this time, I was as healthy as I'd ever been, and the possibility of MS seemed remote. I didn't often think about it, but I never altogether forgot about it either. The little numb spot on my thumb remained, like a footprint or scent marker, just enough to say, *I was here.*

About when I started thinking I might have imagined the whole thing, I happened to get a twenty-four-hour bug accompanied by a high fever. For the day of the fever, the numbness in my thumb became more pronounced, extending to the whole hand. When the fever went away, the numbness receded. This phenomenon was right out of the pre-MRI textbook of diagnostic markers of MS.

From then on, I never dismissed the possibility of having the disease, although I still didn't think about it much. It was like having a sparrow sitting on my shoulder all the time. It weighed nothing, it demanded nothing, but at any moment, it might decide to make a mess on my shirt.

5

THROUGH
A SEA OF MUD

I made only one significant life change with any connection to the possibility of MS: I decided to stop farming.

For several years after the 1995 episode, my then-partner Mary had been urging me to give up farming. Some of the MS books had theorized that stress was a factor in flare-ups, and she worried that the long days of strenuous work in summer heat might be a risk.

Also, I did not have the kind of easygoing temperament that could shrug off the vicissitudes of New England weather. I was a perfectionist about making hay. I *hated* to see it get rained on. I listened to the weather forecast compulsively, and whenever I'd committed to mowing a field, I would be in a state of tension and dread until I had the hay safely dry and in the barn.

Weather forecasting had become remarkably accurate, but New England weather was even more remarkably ornery. All too frequently, the rain that on Sunday was forecast to arrive Wednesday morning would accelerate as it funneled into New England and threaten to arrive Tuesday afternoon, at the precise moment when the hay was dry enough to bale.

More often than not, the day of baling was a race against a darkening western sky. The moment of supreme triumph was to watch the last bale of the day rattle up the hay elevator and into the barn just as the first spatter of rain landed on my head. When we lost the race, I felt an almost physical pain, watching my fluffed windrows of green, fragrant perfection slowly sag and grow sodden in the downpour. Laying down swathes of mown grass under the fickle northeastern sky and counting on two days of sunshine felt like laying myself down and waiting to be kicked. It was foolish to care so much. I repeatedly told myself, "It's just grass, for pity's sake." But I did care, and hence I stressed myself about it, to no useful purpose. (I did make a lot of very beautiful hay, however.)

Other seasons offered their anxieties too. In the winter, I worried about ice that would make footing treacherous for the cows. In the spring, I worried I would be too late finding a cow that needed help calving. In the fall, I worried that I would not have enough customers for my beef. In all seasons, I worried about machinery breaking down. If a calf was sick or a machine broken, I felt faintly on edge until the problem was resolved. The machines were always fixable, but the calves sometimes died, and the trudge into the woods to leave their bodies for the scavengers was a lot worse than a sodden hayfield.

I had a neighbor who never got rattled, no matter what happened on his farm. He had a calm certainty that things would work out, one way or another, and if they didn't, he'd figure out how to deal with it. It was a pleasure to work with him, because he wasted not a speck of energy fretting about things that were out of his control.

Once he brought some new heifers to spend the summer in my pastures. Cows don't like novelty, and two of these heifers got very freaked out by being in a new place. They promptly jumped over several fences and headed off on a mad dash through the countryside. At first, my neighbor and I tried to go after them and head them back, but we soon got reports that they'd been seen two miles away.

It was late in the day. My neighbor said, "Let's leave them be until morning and see what they do."

In the morning, we found the two heifers back inside my pasture with the rest of the herd. They had retraced their two-mile route through strange territory, including jumping back over all the fences, to return to their fellows. Bo-Peep's sheep.

I admired my neighbor's unflappability, but I had never been able to achieve it myself. He was perfectly suited to farming, where both daily activities and overall livelihood are largely governed by factors the farmer can't control. I was forever trying to plan and hated to fail. I loved farming, but it often left me a nervous wreck.

I think my whole family has a propensity toward compulsive planning, trying to control the future. Probably it is a reaction to my father's death. For the two years of his illness, our childhood was shaped by his hospital stays and lung surgeries, and we lived a back-and-forth shuttle between Wyoming and Boston as he was stronger or sicker. After his death came the much longer stretch of years when my mother had to master her own worries and loneliness to keep the family and the ranch functioning.

Many people who met my mother would have said she was fearless. When I was a child, I thought she was too. On the ranch, she was the boss. At parties, she was the magnetic personality who persuaded shy adults to join goofy kid games.

Her Red Angus crusade took her to livestock conferences all over the country, and she often took one or more of her kids with her because she thought it would be as educational as anything at school. I loved roaming the hotel corridors, and I reveled in watching the color TV. (We didn't have a TV in our house because she thought it was the opposite of educational.) More than anything, though, I remember my feeling of awe peeking in the door of a conference room and seeing my mother standing in front of a crowd of skeptical cattlemen, urging them to embrace progress.

When I was older, and she and I conversed as adults, I came to realize that she had spent the decades of my childhood racked by worries about the finances of the ranch, and whether she had the ability to carry on my father's idea, and how she could ever find enough time for her kids. In her later years, she often said to me, "Don't you think the strongest emotion that governs people's lives is fear?"

She was talking about herself. Appearances to the contrary, she was afraid of all sorts of things. In behavior, she was a full-speed-ahead dynamo, but that was her way of getting past her fear: maintaining forward momentum at all times.

Although she could overcome fear, she couldn't get rid of it. It was always there in our family, a presence that no one mentioned directly but all of us felt. The fear of a blind fate that in one stroke could take away the thing you cared about most.

When she came to say prayers with me at bedtime, one part of her prayer always asked blessings on the people she'd lost: Gumbo, her father, who died before I was born; Aunt Judy, her favorite sister, who died in childbirth; Dada, my father. Later, the list would grow to include another of her sisters, who committed suicide, and then her mother. Then, two decades after my father's death, she would lose her daughter, my oldest sister, who collapsed suddenly and died at age thirty-four, possibly from a pulmonary embolism, although the cause of her death was never known for sure.

Only once in my childhood did I hear my mother give voice to fear. She had taken me with her to visit my father's cousin who lived on a ranch many miles down a rough dirt road in southern Montana. Rain had turned stretches of the road to greasy mud, but luckily, we were in a high-clearance, four-wheel-drive vehicle. (My mother was quick to embrace new ideas, and she had bought a Land Rover back around 1960, when four-wheel drive was rare, even on ranches.) It rained while we were visiting, and on the drive home the mud was worse. In the middle of a low place, a quarter-mile stretch of creek bottom, we found ourselves sinking in almost to the axles.

Mud is far more treacherous than snow. If you stop moving, you'll never start again without a tow truck, and this mudhole was a very long walk from help. My mother floored the gas pedal. The Land Rover was spinning and churning and slewing sideways, but somehow she kept us on the road and moving forward, barely. The mud seemed endless, and she had to fight the steering wheel every inch of the way.

Somewhere in the middle of that sea of mud, she started to scream. She kept her grip on the wheel and the gas pedal to the floor and screamed at the top of her lungs. It was a sound I had never heard before and have never heard again, but now that moment feels like an image of my mother in the years after my father's death. Inwardly screaming in terror, but never taking her hands off the wheel or her foot off the gas.

At the time I was conceived, in 1954, my father had already been diagnosed with lung cancer, which was considered incurable. According to my mother, their decision to have another child was intentional. She said she had wanted to give him motivation for the struggle that lay ahead, as if the six kids he already had weren't motivation enough. I have to think it was a colossal act of denial by both of them, and I have been favorably disposed toward denial ever since.

In the case of my MS symptoms, I suppose that putting them out of my mind was akin to my mother keeping her foot on the gas or my father deciding to have another child: don't stop living until you're actually dead.

I think it is almost impossible not to be in denial about our own death or disability. We see ourselves from the inside, and it is hard to imagine an inner state of being altogether different from our actual experience.

I can picture my body in a wheelchair or a coffin or, for that matter, on the stage at Carnegie Hall playing the piano. But that picture seen from the outside doesn't feel real, because it doesn't correspond to the way I experience myself. I can tell myself, rationally, that a certain event

might happen, and I can write my will or take other practical steps to prepare. But on some level, I won't feel the
reality of it.

It is easier to be a clear-eyed realist about another
person, because there is a correspondence between one's
imagining of possibilities and one's actual experience.
Both of them happen from the outside. If I picture a friend
in a wheelchair, I see the image from the same perspective
as I see the friend now.

Perhaps that is why Mary worried about the stress of
farm work more than I did. At the end of a day of haying,
she could see how tired I looked, with my clothing soaked
in sweat and my skin flecked with bits of hay. She was the
one who listened to me fretting about the weather, chastis-
ing myself for failing to save a calf, and cursing the safety
shields that made it a finger-pinching trial to grease the
U-joints on the mower. For her, it was a shorter step from
the stress she could see in front of her to the picture of
me somehow disabled. I just felt strong and capable and
couldn't imagine myself feeling otherwise.

I did finally decide to stop farming, but not primarily
out of concern for my health. Mostly I wanted more time
for other things.

I sold my mother cows a few at a time over a period
of months, fortunately to other breeders rather than for
slaughter. I kept my favorite half-Jersey cow Giselle and a
couple of my Red Angus heifers so that I could continue
to raise beef for home use. The equipment went all at once
on a bright, sunny day in August. The auction lasted barely
an hour and was a rousing success, perhaps a payoff for my
perfectionism about maintenance, as a lot of the machinery brought more money than I had paid for it.

I kept one tractor, an indestructible thirty-five-year-old workhorse John Deere 2020 with an oversize bucket loader and a permanent black protective coating composed of oil, grease, hydraulic fluid, coolant, dust, and chaff. By the end of the day, the rest of my equipment had been hauled away to other farms.

The next day, walking around the empty farmstead, I was in a state of grief. Even now, twenty years later, I have a tactile memory of every single machine I worked with: the rattle of worn gears in the tedder, the stiffness of its adjustment crank, the weight of each hitch, the trick to backing the angled wheels of the rake, the strenuous heave to spin the starter wheel on the old motor baler I kept as a backup, the wonderfully light steering on the 2440 tractor, the exact place to wedge a block of wood before loosening the blade bolts on the disc mower, and the many dozens of grease nipples on everything. Especially I remember myself on the seat of the 2440, looking back at my towed caravan of baler and hay wagon, watching my nephew on the wagon alternately stacking the bales and playing games of dodgeball with them as they flew off the spinning belts of the bale thrower.

6

FROM MAYBE
TO YES

Not long after I stopped farming, I started learning to contradance.

When I was in elementary school, one of our neighbors had led evenings of dance lessons at the community clubhouse a few miles from our ranch. The clubhouse was a beautiful old log building with a smooth wood floor, a massive fieldstone fireplace for atmosphere, and coal stoves at each end of the room for heat. The neighbor taught a variety of dances—polka, varsoviana, butterfly waltz, circle mixers, and the basics of square dance—to a crowd of all ages, people from the ranches up and down the valley. My favorite moment was dancing the butterfly with my best friend and her father. Her father was a big man, and as my friend and I took turns hooking elbows with him, he could easily whirl us off our feet.

In college, I had loved to dance, in the random-gyra-tion-to-rock-and-Motown style of campus dances in the 1970s, but after graduation I stopped, in large part because I'd come out as gay. At that age, I was far too shy to make a public display of my otherness on a floor filled with straight couples.

By 2002, it was less of a statement to dance with another woman. My new partner Ruth was a folk dancer, and I leapt at the chance to join her in the sociable walking figures of New England contradance. Although I spent my first few dances in deep concentration, working to learn the figures, I was also on a high, whirling around the floor, propelled by the crazy-fast fiddling and stop-for-nothing rhythm of the music.

My mother was delighted that I was dancing, although she was a bit dismissive of contradancing as "too slow" compared to square dancing. She and my father had been avid square dancers, and, among the infinity of things she had lost with his death, she had lost her dance partner. In her determined way, she had continued to go to dances, but in Wyoming at that time it was bleak to arrive without a partner. The culture of square dance was to "dance with the one that brung ya," and in many cases even a square of four couples would dance the entire evening together. Unless a man had arrived without a partner—an uncommon event—my mother could only hope that some of the ladies might want a rest when their husbands didn't so that she would be invited to dance. I often wished that her neighborhood had had contradances, where the culture is to mix with partners around the room, and singles are not left stranded on the sidelines.

Around the time I gained some confidence about dancing, a friend upped the ante on learning new things. She remembered my having said I would like to learn to play an instrument someday and offered to give me her brother's old student clarinet, which was sitting abandoned in her closet. Playing an instrument was one of many things I'd said I'd like to do someday, with little expectation that I would follow through. Now I was being offered a clarinet, an instrument I loved. It was a put up or shut up moment, and I said yes.

My friend showed me how to wet the reed and clamp it with the ligature, and how to place my lips on the mouthpiece. She explained that the reed makes sound in the same way a blade of grass makes sound if you stretch it between your steepled thumbs and blow air across it through the gap. The gap must be right, the tension right, the airstream right, or the grass will not sing.

Following her directions, I tried blowing through the mouthpiece. The only sound was a whoosh of air. I tried some more, adjusting my lip, adjusting my breath, getting nothing but sighs and wheezes of unproductive wind. Then, suddenly, my lip found the sweet spot, and the reed let out a wail. That was all it took. With just that one wavering untuned note, roughly a high C, the clarinet had me hooked.

The instrument came with some easy Yamaha instruction books, as well as a terrifying inch-thick book of densely packed exercises by somebody named Klosé. (Klosé, I later learned, is the brewer's yeast of the clarinet world, an object of devotion to some players and loathing to others, but unquestionably good for you if you can choke him down.) Teaching myself to play, I stuck to the Yamaha books and their repertoire of familiarity—"Danny Boy," Sousa marches, "Sweet Betsy from Pike," and hits from *The Nutcracker.*

I loved every minute of practice. Dancing to the music of others, I had thought the high was as good as it gets, but as I found music starting to emerge from my own breath and fingers, even the silliest and simplest of tunes, I felt as if I had embarked on an enterprise whose joys and aspirations had no upper limit. Best of all, since Ruth played the cello at a recreational level, I could hope that I might someday learn the clarinet well enough for us to play together.

By then, Ruth had moved in with me, and we were making plans for a civil union ceremony the following spring. More than eight years had passed since the 1995 episode of neurological symptoms. Even the patch of numbness on my thumb, my little reminder spot, had gone away. More and more, I thought the symptoms might have been a passing oddity. I did keep up my dietary regimen, however.

The year 2004 would be a watershed on many fronts. In May, Ruth and I celebrated our civil union at a local Girl Scout camp overlooking a large pond. We chose the month to avoid the busiest seasons for my brothers on the ranch. We chose the day to fit the schedule of a caller and a band we particularly loved, and the venue had to have a large wooden dance floor. (It went without saying that we would have a contradance.) When the day came, friends decorated the camp dining hall with quantities of lilacs and sorted through the orange and blue plastic chairs to leave only the blue ones at the tables arranged for dinner.

Except for one niece who was in the last month of pregnancy, my entire family attended the celebration— my mother, my five siblings and their spouses, my sister's widower and his wife, and my other seven nieces and nephews, some with spouses. Before the ceremony, we all gathered on the lawn outside the hall and perched on some slightly wobbly bleachers to have pictures taken. Those photographs of all of us are the last I have in which we are all together and all smiling. A year later, my mother would barely survive a stroke, and with her resulting loss of capacities, a host of subterranean resentments and hostilities would surface and fracture the family.

In June, my first grandniece was born. She was given the name Sarah, the name of my mother and sister and several earlier forebears. In September, Ruth's father, Mike, died at age ninety. He passed rather quickly, from pneumonia following a heart attack. Ruth and her mother had a couple of days with him in the hospital, saying goodbyes, before he slipped into a coma. On the last day, when he was unconscious, one of their friends brought her violin to his room to play him to his rest.

In October, I turned fifty and, after decades of agonized fandom, saw the Boston Red Sox finally win the World Series. Ruth and I joked that maybe her father had been able to pull some strings.

My own father had been a Red Sox fan also, and my mother liked to tell a story about him from a time late in his illness. It was September, and she and my uncle and aunt were sitting with him in his hospital room. He was lying with his eyes closed, not responding to their conversation. His skin was bluish, and they thought he might be on the point of slipping away. Then he began to speak, and they quickly leaned closer to hear what he was saying, in case these were his final words.

"Bravo," he said, and then, "Ted Williams hit a home run . . . that's good."

Only then did they notice the radio on the bedside table, next to his ear. It was playing at low volume, tuned to the ball game.

As he was speaking, some pinkness returned to his skin, and soon after that, his strength picked up a bit. He was able to leave the hospital and have another couple of months at home before he died.

In the weeks between my father-in-law Mike's death and the Red Sox victory, my neurological symptoms reappeared. The numbness and tingling were more widespread, from my feet and legs all the way up to my hands, and included a new feature, the sensation that I had a tight rubber band around my torso at the level of my diaphragm.

The rubber band sensation was a tactile hallucination. I could breathe perfectly normally. In fact, as far as I could tell, all of my motor function was normal. The numbness did have one practical effect, however. I couldn't feel the keys of my new clarinet well enough to keep playing.

Soon after the onset of symptoms, Ruth and I joined some friends on a car-camping trip in the desert in Utah. The trip had been planned long before, and apart from the weird nerve sensations, I felt fit and strong, so we went ahead. We talked about whether to tell our friends about the symptoms and agreed we wouldn't, unless the symptoms got worse. I didn't want our friends to spend their whole vacation worrying about me.

Both of us were a bit concerned about the desert heat, and Ruth made me promise that I wouldn't push myself in the compulsive way that I usually did. For once in my life, I would take it easy and be content with a few miles of hiking each day, unless it was cool, in which case I could sneak in a run.

The trip had no detectable effect on my health, except to make me very happy. In the daytime, we explored the carved-rock landscape of slot canyons and stone arches. In the evening, we sat around a campfire, feasting and talking. Before flying home, we spent a night in Las Vegas, a splash of noise and cheerful garishness that heightened the effect of the previous week in the company of sinewy vegetation, clear air, rocks, and silence.

When we got home from the desert, I made an appointment to see a doctor.

Without the civil union, I might not have had a family doctor to see. Dr. Hale had retired, and most of the private family practices in our region were full and not taking new patients. Luckily, Ruth had an established relationship with a doctor in a small group practice, and he let me "marry in" to his patient list.

Dr. Clement was easy to talk to, low key and relaxed. He knew a lot, and we could joke with him, a happy combination. He also tolerated my peppering him with questions, even those that sprang from idle curiosity rather than practical necessity.

Dr. Clement confirmed that my symptoms might be MS. To know for sure, I should have MRIs and see a neurologist. As far as which neurologist, he said I had various choices. I could go back to Dr. Sage, at the medical center, and he would probably see me the soonest, since I'd seen him before. Alternatively, I could try to see a different doctor at the medical center, one of a neurology subgroup that specialized in MS. A third option was a private neurology clinic for which he had high regard. He said I might want to get an opinion from both the medical center and the clinic, because now there were medications available and different doctors followed different schools of thought.

I told him that, although I had liked Dr. Sage, I thought it made sense to consult a doctor who specialized in MS. We agreed that I would also consult a doctor at the private clinic. The first step, however, was for one of the neurologists to order the MRIs and get them scheduled.

As had happened with the previous episode, I had to wait a couple of months for the MRIs. By the time I got them, my symptoms had mostly vanished. My legs and torso were normal, and the rubber band around my diaphragm was gone. I still had residual numbness and prickling in my hands, but it had diminished enough that I could resume practicing the clarinet. In a gesture of optimism, I found a music teacher and began taking lessons for the first time.

My symptoms had lasted for a few weeks in September and October. I had the MRIs at the beginning of January. The follow-up neurology appointments were scheduled for February. Later I would have reason to be glad that the system worked so slowly, but while I was waiting to learn the results, I chafed at the delay.

I suppose I imagined that I would sit down in an exam room, and the doctor would explain to me what the MRIs

had found, good or bad. What actually happened was perhaps more typical of our health-care complex, in which
astounding technical sophistication and superb practitioners are stuck in a Rube Goldberg contraption, linked
together by clankingly inefficient systems of communication, administration, and payment.

Late in January, I got a call from the receptionist at
the small private clinic. She said she was calling about the
schedule for my appointment to discuss my MS diagnosis.
I said, "Oh?" and then, when I'd caught my breath, "So the
MRIs definitely showed MS?"

Now she was the one who said, "Oh." And then, "You
didn't know?"

I bit back the urge to snap, *How would I know? No one
told me they had the results back.*

Perhaps I should have been calling the neurologists'
offices every day to ask. Perhaps that was the only way to
get information, but I hadn't wanted to bug them. It's a
catch-22. The doctors are too busy to call or send a letter with test results, and if the patient keeps calling to ask
about them, it makes the doctors even busier.

Instead, the receptionist became the unwitting bearer
of bad news, with no chance to prepare the ground. It
shouldn't have mattered how I learned my diagnosis
because, really, it was very old news. I'd been living with
the possibility of MS for eleven years. But it turned out
there was a big difference, psychologically, between maybe
and yes.

At the time, I was annoyed, but in retrospect the inci-
dent came to seem comic. The receptionist was more cha-
grined than I was, and the mix-up certainly wasn't her
fault. It wasn't any other single person's fault either. It's just

the way our system often functions when it engages the bigger gears.

I would encounter a similar lurch and grind in the gears when I arrived at my medical center appointment. The only reason I opted not to go back to Dr. Sage was to see an MS specialist, but somewhere along the way, that piece of the plan did not get communicated. The new doctor to whom I was referred was not an MS specialist. I could only hope that the time was long enough and the world busy enough that Dr. Sage would never know about this referral. I would have no chance to explain to him that the change from one nonspecialist to another nonspecialist was just a screwup in the system and not due to any dissatisfaction with his care.

The good news about all the long delays was that I had plenty of time to think. After I learned of my diagnosis, weeks passed before I saw a neurologist. In the interval I was able to do some research on the new drugs that were available.

There were two types that had been on the market for a number of years. One type was interferon, which worked by suppressing production of immune cells. There were a couple of brand names, Avonex and Betaseron, made by different manufacturers. The other type, made by a single manufacturer, was called Copaxone. It worked by trying to block immune cells from attacking myelin. Both types were given by injection, daily or weekly, and promised to reduce the frequency of flare-ups by about 30 percent, averaged over a large study group. The drugs had various side effects, such as flu symptoms, which were cheerfully described as "manageable with Tylenol."

Coincidentally, even though the two types of drug worked by completely different mechanisms and were produced by different manufacturers, they cost almost exactly the same amount, about $1,400 per month. They were intended to be a lifelong treatment, unless something better came along.

As I was in the midst of this research on existing drugs, my brother-in-law John sent me a news bulletin about a brand-new MS drug that had been fast-tracked for approval by the FDA. The drug had originally been scheduled for a two-year clinical trial before it could be approved, but after the first year of the trial, the results looked so promising that the FDA had gone ahead and approved it. It was called Tysabri, or natalizumab, and it was one of a relatively new type of drugs known as monoclonal antibody drugs. It was given monthly by IV infusion, and its preliminary results indicated it reduced the frequency of flare-ups by about 60 percent.

After reading about the various drugs online, I went back to the medical center library to see if the other types of information I had found there nine years earlier had been updated or expanded. Had anything new been learned about the causes of the disease or the possible benefits of changes in lifestyle?

What I found instead was that all the books that had been there nine years earlier were gone and had not been replaced with updated information. The medical center library no longer had any books for the general public about epidemiology, lifestyle studies, or anything else to do with MS. Apparently, now that pharmaceutical treatments were available, the other kinds of information were not thought to be of interest.

7

THE RISK
MADE VISIBLE

The first of my appointments was at the small private neurology clinic. The building was pleasant and the atmosphere friendly. I was shown into a spacious office with light streaming in the window.

The first person to see me was a physician's assistant, a warm middle-aged woman who radiated concern for her patients. She said she had worked with many, many people with MS, and she grew almost tearful, saying how happy she was that they finally had a new drug to offer that might make a significant difference.

Explaining how the treatment process worked, she said I would come in once a month to be hooked up for an IV infusion, rather like chemotherapy. She reassured me that although the drug was very expensive, something like $2,800 per month, it would probably be covered by my insurance, since I had Blue Cross. If my insurance didn't cover it, the drug company had a program to subsidize part of the cost.

At some point in the course of my conversation with the PA, the neurologist came in to join us. Dr. Avanti was vigorous, articulate, and personable, and his manner suggested that he was a forward thinker, quick to embrace progress. Neither he nor the PA conveyed any doubt that the new drug was the way to go. The clinical trial indicated that it was twice as effective as the older drugs, so why would anyone go with the older drugs?

I demurred a bit. The trial had only lasted a year. To be included in the trial, patients must have had at least two flare-ups in the two previous years, a rate nine times more frequent than mine. How could Dr. Avanti be certain that the results were applicable to me when the pattern of my symptoms was so different from the people in the study?

Also, the treatment was complex, inconvenient, and expensive. It had side effects. My symptoms were very mild. Was it worth it?

Dr. Avanti was emphatic. The whole point of the drug was that you take it *before* you have serious symptoms, to reduce the frequency of flare-ups and therefore the speed of deterioration. It was ideal that I was so "early" in the course of the disease.

I asked if there were any studies that compared the effectiveness of drugs to the effectiveness of diet and other lifestyle changes. I thought I already knew the answer, and Dr. Avanti confirmed my surmise. No such studies existed, as far as he knew. My question did start us on a pleasant chat about the epidemiology of the disease, and he mentioned the curious case of the Faroe Islands.

At the end of the appointment, I had not come to any decision about treatment. I said I wanted to hear the opinion of the medical center neurologist first. The PA gave me literature about the new drug to take home and read. Her concern was palpable. Somehow she had to persuade me to accept their help. In her view, my future depended on it.

When I went to my appointment at the medical center, the atmosphere was quite different. Everyone was pleasant, but, unlike the staff at the private clinic, they did not greet me with a gracious welcome as if I were a valued customer. The place was busy and businesslike. I was led through a windowless rabbit warren of offices to a small, spartan room, also windowless. The lighting wasn't dim, but somehow it felt dim.

The neurologist came in soon after, carrying a laptop. Dr. Blunt was compact and brisk, with short dark hair and a slight German accent.

The conversation did not start well. After introductions, I said, "I understand you're part of the group that specializes in MS."

"No, I'm not in that group," she said, "but my knowledge of MS is completely adequate for your situation."

Her tone was a bit irritable, and I couldn't tell if she felt I had impugned her knowledge and was offended or she was impatient that someone whose case was unremarkable would expect a specialist.

I muddled out an explanation that I wasn't questioning her capability, but I'd been expecting a referral to an MS specialist, because that was the only reason I'd changed doctors. I said I didn't want the neurology department to think I was dissatisfied with her colleague. We quickly came to a couple of points of agreement: some wires must have gotten crossed somewhere in the referral process, and it really didn't matter if I saw a specialist. After that, the conversation went better.

She opened her laptop, which turned out to be effectively her office. She simply carried it with her to whatever exam room was available for her next appointment. Her manner had none of Dr. Avanti's polish. She was Dragnet, "just the facts, ma'am," and I liked that. The first thing she did was to pull up my MRIs and put them on the screen so that I could look at them. She could not have found a shorter path into my heart.

She displayed the brain MRI first and pointed at two tiny white spots. "You have more than one lesion. That confirms the diagnosis. But these are not the ones that worry me."

She closed the brain scan and opened the scan of my spine. I could see the elongated S curve from the base of the skull down to the lower back and the dark line of the spinal cord running down the chain of vertebrae. She zeroed in on the neck and pointed at a large white blob on the spinal cord. "This is the one that worries me."

She then proceeded to explain her worry, although in essence I had understood it the moment I saw the pictures. The brain is large and has a large amount of reserve capacity. If one bit of tissue gets damaged, the brain often can rewire itself to use a different part and not lose any function. But the spine does not have any backup capacity. If the lesion in my cervical spine went bad, it could affect function anywhere in my body from the neck down.

I had read about the possible effects of MS. I knew that relapses were unpredictable and were likely to become more damaging. I knew that in bad cases they could progress to incontinence, spasticity, vision loss, and even paralysis. But this knowledge had been conveyed to me in words, which kept it safely abstract. My actual symptoms were so mild and my relapses so infrequent that it was easy to think my risk must be small.

Now Dr. Blunt confronted me with a palpable image of the risk, a lesion eating away at my spinal cord. The lesion had reached a point at which it caused lasting symptoms: the numbness in my hands. If it flared again, it would almost certainly leave more significant symptoms.

There are many ways one can figuratively have a sword hanging by a thread over one's head. Death hangs there for everyone. But that white blob in my neck brought the figurative image much too close to the here and now, the allegorical sword made flesh. At any moment, my misguided T cells could launch an attack and take another bite out of my spinal cord. Clearly, the goal was to avoid another attack, because the next bite might sever some important function.

I asked Dr. Blunt what she advised. In principle, she said the same thing as Dr. Avanti; I should go on medication, and it was important to start immediately, because the medications worked by reducing the incidence of flare-ups. She said I could try either interferon or Copaxone. Their effectiveness was similar, and it was just a question of which one my system tolerated better.

I told her that Dr. Avanti had recommended the newer drug, Tysabri, and asked her what she thought. She said she didn't recommend it because it was too new, and there was not yet sufficient data. She said that in most cases the medical center leaned toward caution in its approach and preferred treatments with a track record.

After my appointment at the private clinic, I had been quite swept up in their enthusiasm for the new drug. Much as I hate taking medications of any kind, their urgency made me start to consider how the program of monthly infusions could fit into my life. MS is a frightening prospect, and the clinic staff had been positively bursting with hopefulness.

Thinking back on their attitude, I realize that medical people who specialize in chronic diseases like MS must get a very skewed experience. The type of patient they see the most is the one who is doing badly, so their desire to take action and help is understandably very urgent. They may hear indirectly about patients who do well without intervention, but they don't *see* those people all the time. Probably I needn't have worried about offending Dr. Sage by changing doctors, because he had not seen me in nine years and very likely had forgotten I existed.

Dr. Blunt's caution was much closer to my native outlook, and when she voiced her skepticism, I felt as if a bubble of fantasy had been popped. I might still consider the new drug, but I would choose a treatment on the basis of data, practicalities, and my own body and not be swayed by the personal enthusiasm of the practitioners.

Her skepticism also reawakened my resistance to the idea of drugs in general. I raised the same question I had at the clinic. Was the data from two-year studies applicable to a case with only one flare-up in nine years? Given the mildness of the symptoms, were the side effects of treatment worth it? I was doing very well on my dietary program. My body was generally very healthy. Why mess with it?

I said I could see a lot of reasons not to go on medication and asked her if that would be a reasonable decision. She said, "It's your choice, but you'll be taking a risk."

Then I said, "Ten years ago, there weren't any medications. What would you have told me about the likely course of the disease back then?"

She said, "I'd have told you it will get worse."

8

CALCULATING
THE ODDS

I went home to think about the information from the two neurologists. Trying to come to a decision, I was in a mental tug-of-war. On the one hand, although the doctors disagreed about which medication I should take, they were in agreement that I should take *something*. On the other hand, I hated taking drugs.

For the most part, I thought my body had served me well. Apart from this little quirk that it occasionally started chewing on itself, my immune system functioned admirably. I got sick rarely and recovered quickly. The idea of putting hobbles on my immune system to slow its attack on my nervous system was a very mixed prospect.

Part of my reluctance stemmed from the medical literature itself. I had read about how the various drugs worked, and it was clear that none of them targeted the cause of the illness. They were not like antibiotics that kill the organism that is making you sick or taking vitamin C as a remedy for scurvy.

The cause of MS was still unknown. Doctors didn't know what made my immune system start attacking my own tissue. Because they didn't know the cause, they couldn't treat the cause. However, they did know the agent of the disease, the T cells of the immune system, so the only strategy available was to throw up roadblocks between the T cells and their wrongheaded target in the nerves. Although the treatments tried to limit the effect of these roadblocks, they caused collateral damage. The frequency of flu symptoms as a side effect showed that the drugs affected immune function in ways other than their intended purpose.

I was strongly of the mindset "if it ain't broke, don't fix it." I'd been running in the same model of running shoes for twenty years without suffering any injuries, so why would I start buying a different model? For years I used a clothespin to wedge the Start button on my lovely analog dial toaster oven, postponing the day when I would have to endure all the annoying digital buttons and beeps of the newer ones.

Whether it was laziness, thrift, or pathology, I wasn't the only one in my family with this attitude. When my sister and her husband moved into a retirement community, the house they left behind still had the same metal-door kitchen cabinets it had had when they moved into it as a young married couple.

In the matter of my health, I didn't feel "broken" most of the time. I had to remind myself that my immune system did have a problem, and the drugs were supposed to help. But when I did the math on the potential benefit of the medications, I was not immediately won over.

The drug promised a 30 percent reduction in frequency of flare-ups on average. If that number held up in my case, the nine-and-a-half-year interval since my last flare would be expected to improve to thirteen years before my next one. In other words, I would have to be on the drug for more than a decade before I would have a clue if it was helping me, and in the meantime, it had side effects. In a decade, I would meet lots of other threats from which the immune system protected me. So what were the odds?

The doctors had wider experience with the disease than I did, and they thought the best approach was intervention. However, I had more experience with my own body, and I wasn't sure. I had mentioned my dietary regimen to both of them and asked if there was any "scientific," as opposed to "anecdotal," information on the subject. The answer was no. There were no studies in which a statistically meaningful group of people had done what I had done.

Neither of the neurologists seemed very interested in my anecdotal experience. I had the feeling that they didn't want to encourage my belief in my regimen, because they were afraid I would be like the people who went off to Mexico to pursue herbal remedies instead of following a proven chemotherapy protocol for deadly cancer. From their perspective, it was vital to persuade me to take the drugs, for my own good and also to defend the whole principle of the scientific method from the quacks who peddled untested hope to desperate people.

In their minds my diet was not a treatment. But in my mind it was a treatment. In my statistically meaningless study group of one, I had changed my diet, and my remission period had improved more than sixfold, going from a year and a half to more than nine years. That was twice as good as the fancy new drug and four times as good as the old ones, with no negative side effects. If it had been a drug that gave me this result, the doctors would have said I should keep taking it. But it wasn't a drug, and it hadn't been studied.

I was never in doubt that I would continue with my eating habits. The question was whether I should also take a drug and, if so, which one. I was leaning toward Dr. Blunt's philosophy, trying one of the older drugs. If it had bad side effects, I could stop. But I wasn't very happy about the idea.

This was the moment when my course was changed by the slowness of the medical wheels. I had waited months for the MRI and weeks more after that for the follow-up appointments. In the days after my appointments, I was balanced on a seesaw of indecision.

But in the time that had elapsed in my personal medical process, time had also elapsed in the ongoing clinical trial of Tysabri. In the week when I was due to make my decision, a story about the trial hit the national news. The drug had been abruptly yanked from the market because of an infrequent but unacceptable side effect. A couple of trial patients had died.

The cause of death was a rare brain virus, to which the drug had apparently made the patients more susceptible. The trial group was not very large, a few hundred including the controls who weren't getting the drug, so a couple of untimely deaths were very significant.

My first reaction was a nod of gratitude to Dr. Blunt for her caution. As I went on reading, though, I discovered the story was more complex than just a failure of Tysabri. From the point of view of future treatment, it was a good news/bad news situation. The good news was that Tysabri might not be altogether bad. The bad news was that one of the older drugs might not be altogether benign.

It turned out that the clinical trial had three different groups: the patients on Tysabri, the control group on an interferon drug, and a third group who were on a combination therapy of Tysabri and interferon. The patients who died belonged to the third group. It was the combination of the two drugs that was fatal.

The conclusion drawn by the medical system was simply that the two drugs should not be used in combined therapy. After some further testing, Tysabri would be returned to the market on that basis. It could not be used on patients who also took interferon. Each drug taken as a single therapy was considered to be safe enough that its benefits outweighed its risks.

The conclusion I drew for myself was somewhat different. To my eye, the trial result was more evidence that both of the drugs had effects on the immune system that went beyond their intended therapeutic target. Only when the effects were combined did they quickly become fatal, but that didn't mean the effects were negligible individually. To say that singly the drugs were harmless would be like saying it's harmless to remove one of the lug nuts from your wheel hub because the wheel won't actually fall off unless it has lost two lug nuts.

For the people in the clinical trials, who typically suffered annual relapses, the modest risks of single therapy probably were outweighed by the benefits. In ten years, such people could expect to reduce their number of relapses from ten down to seven, on average. But for me to experience the same amount of improvement, from ten relapses down to seven, I would have to be on the drug for ninety years, or until I was 140 years old.

I did not have a blanket objection to drugs. When I got a bacterial infection, I took antibiotics. If I were to get a deadly cancer for which chemotherapy offered a 30 percent chance of cure, I would take the chemotherapy. With the cancer, the choice would be between certain death and a 30 percent chance of survival, and the odds would be worth the cost. With MS, though, the future was a wide range of possibility from good health to complete disability, with or without drugs. The drugs merely promised a modest reduction in the speed at which my future would arrive.

As I was trying to make up my mind, I often appealed to Ruth for a reality check. In varying ways, I asked her, "Would I be crazy not to do what the doctors say?"

She never urged me, in either direction. She had listened patiently as I reasoned out loud, and perhaps she shared my skepticism. Or perhaps she just knew I was stubborn.

It was not that she didn't worry about me or give advice in general. She routinely urged me to be careful driving on snowy roads or reminded me to jog on the side of the road facing traffic. On the topic of MS, though, I think she knew I needed to believe in whatever path I chose, so it had to be my decision. If she had asked me to take the drugs for her sake, for her peace of mind, I probably would have done so, but she did not ask that.

In the end, the news about the Tysabri trial tipped my seesaw back the other way. I decided to do what Dr. Blunt described as "taking a chance." I decided to do without the drugs.

This was not an irrevocable decision. I put it in the form of a bargain, with myself, with people I loved, with my doctors. For the moment, I would not take any drugs. But if I had another relapse relatively soon, within a couple of years, then I would try taking one of them.

This decision was based partly on the pure mathematics of the ratio between my relapse rate and the predicted benefit of the drug. But it was also based on my knowledge of myself, which was something clinical trials couldn't measure, and the neurologists couldn't learn about in a half-hour appointment.

All doctors learn about the placebo effect. Some of them seem to view it as a nuisance, like friction in a physics problem, a factor that scientific studies have to filter out before the study results are meaningful. Other doctors see it as a tool in their toolbox. Both Dr. Hale and Dr. Clement, my family doctors, were in the latter category, and they seemed to understand that to use placebos effectively the doctor has to know the patient. One patient's placebo is another patient's poison.

For me in this particular case, forgoing the drug was the placebo. It was the path that would harness my own mind most effectively to promote my own health. I disliked drugs, and if I took one, some part of me would always be resisting it. If I chose not to take a drug, every ounce of my will would be directed toward a single purpose: to stay healthy so that I could continue to justify not taking a drug.

I had seen the blob on my spinal cord. I recognized the risk. Time would tell if my decision was foolish, but it felt right to me.

9

THE WATERWORKS

In one respect, getting MS was like realizing I was gay. Before I came out, I had known exactly one person who was gay, one of my college professors. My admiration for him helped me break through the denial in my head.

He was a living refutation of the attitude that had surrounded me growing up, the universal but unspoken belief that gay people were weird. I didn't think I was weird, and as long as I believed gay people were weird, I assumed I wasn't one of them. But my professor was not weird. He was marvelous. He was funny and ebullient and made you feel that Shakespeare was talking about exactly the same human puzzle you and your friends had been talking about last night at dinner, only with more memorable words. Even though I was in no way like him and certainly not marvelous in the way he was, his existence made it no longer unthinkable that I could be gay.

In my last year of college, I came out. And suddenly, after twenty-two years knowing no one who was gay, I felt as though gay people were appearing from the woodwork. A classmate I'd known for three years told me he was gay and was launching forth into a brave new world of gorgeous men. (Two years later, AIDS hit the news. I had lost touch with him by then and don't know if he survived his launch.) Soon after that, another college friend confessed she was gay and we mutually made a pass at each other, though the connection didn't last. I became acquainted with two of my cousins, one of whom was gay and the other bisexual. And so it continued. Everywhere I went, I met people who were gay. The change was like the difference between my ears hearing an undifferentiated twitter of birds and a bird-watching enthusiast hearing the distinct song of each species. My mind was now tuned to noticing.

The same thing happened with MS. Before I had it myself, I did not know anyone who had it. My first long-term partner sometimes mentioned a family friend who had MS, but that was my only personal connection to the disease, a secondhand story about someone who knew someone. And I had heard of Jacqueline du Pré.

Then I had my flare-up in 1995 and began to take an interest in the disease. That same summer, as I was beginning my experiment with diet, my softball team was standing around one evening, drinking beer after a game on one of the small-town ball fields in our league. In the course of conversation, our tough and ferociously disciplined catcher mentioned that she was having problems with her eyesight.

"I've lost half my field of vision," she said. "It's like something covering part of my eye."

As she described more details, I blurted out, "That sounds like multiple sclerosis."

She looked startled, but said MS was one possibility the doctors had mentioned, and she would be getting MRIs. Soon after that, her diagnosis was confirmed.

As time passed, more friends and acquaintances showed up with MS. The wife of my closest friend from college. The sister of my closest friend from high school. The stepson of my neighbor. An ex-girlfriend's nephew. It wasn't a sudden new epidemic of the disease. It was that people were more likely to mention cases they knew about, and when the topic came up by chance, it caught my attention. The effect was to make me feel that MS was rather commonplace.

In 2005, when my diagnosis was confirmed, the people I knew with MS had an experience similar to mine. None of them were incapacitated by the disease. Some took medication. Some chose not to. We didn't see one another often enough to compare experiences in detail, but none of us wanted to dwell on the subject.

I did not join any public support groups for MS, in the same way that I had generally not sought out social groups centered on gayness. Both things were incidental circumstances in my life. I'd already learned that sharing the trait of being gay did not mean that another person and I had anything else in common. We might, or we might not. If I was seeking kinship, I had better odds in a group of gardeners or book lovers whose gender proclivities could be anything.

With MS, I did consider going to a group, mostly because of my scientific curiosity about the disease. A group might be a source of anecdotal data that didn't get recorded in studies. The big problem was time. Getting married at age fifty had given me a whole new circle of attachments without adding any hours to the day, and I already had trouble keeping up.

I also worried I would embarrass myself in a meeting, because I suffered from a maddening inability to stop myself from weeping at inopportune moments for the smallest of reasons. I couldn't ever talk to anyone about the 2004 baseball playoff series in which the Red Sox came back to beat the Yankees after being behind three games to zero, because when I got to game 4, when the score was tied and I turned off the TV and went to bed because I couldn't bear to watch the final loss, and then described waking up in the morning to discover the Red Sox had won the game, I would start to sob. It was ridiculous. I couldn't stop myself, and there was often no proportion to the importance of the event.

I was as liable to cry talking about the Denver Broncos finally winning the Super Bowl as I was talking about my sister's death. Sitting at the breakfast table, I couldn't tell Ruth about a newspaper story in which a passerby risked his life to pull somebody out of a burning car. I couldn't stand up in a group to talk about anything I really cared about, and I definitely couldn't talk about a dog dying, not even a dog who only existed in a book.

Physical disability was a hypothetical prospect, but functionally I had a handicap here and now. At town meetings, it kept me silent in the back row, seething rather than voicing an opinion, because I knew if I went to the microphone to talk, I was likely to choke up. I'd seen other speakers weep disproportionately at the microphone, and the misplaced emotion didn't help their cause. Tears during a funeral eulogy rouse empathy, but tears during a policy discussion are just embarrassing.

So I was wary of talking about MS in any public setting for fear that the waterworks might leak. People would think I was crying because I was terribly distraught about my health situation. They wouldn't understand that I could get equally choked up describing a dramatic play in a football game or trying to explain what I loved about a particular contradance. There were times when this was a terrific impediment to normal conversation.

In the summer of 2005, a few months after my diagnosis was confirmed, some friends of ours from New Orleans were due to spend a month at our house. Ruth had known Tom and Tracey for twenty years and opened her house to them and their two kids every summer. I had married into the connection. Whereas Ruth and I were quiet in our habits, our friends were a lively, enterprising, talkative bunch, and their younger child was sixteen, so arguments were part of the daily routine. Unlike Ruth's prior house, where their entire family had camped in her living room, our house did have a guestroom, but the six of us were still living very much family-style. Along with coziness and camaraderie, there was a certain amount of discussion about who splashed water around like a duck at the kitchen sink and who else might have failed to make a note on the grocery list after finishing the jar of mayonnaise.

During their previous visits, I hadn't mentioned the MS. The 1995 episode was far in the past, and I wasn't certain I had the disease. With this recent scare, Ruth and

I decided we should talk about it. We knew the stress of merging divergent lifestyles was not all on our side. Our friends felt they were creeping around like mice, and they still heard us grumble about the lack of peace.

We all sat down at the table in the open-plan kitchen and dining room, which was the place we spent most of our free time. I was dreading the conversation, because it felt so self-dramatizing. Even during the flare-up, I had been quite healthy. Now my only complaint was that my hands felt a kind of electric buzz when I washed dishes or filed my nails. Anything truly bad was still theoretical.

I began to explain the particular reason I was concerned about stress. Just as I'd feared, when I reached the point where I had to bring out the words to talk about MS, I started to cry. I was furious, but also trapped. Because I was crying, I couldn't speak clearly enough to explain that my tears were just a stupid hormone malfunction that was like a piece of burnt toast setting off the sprinkler system in the whole building.

I worried that our friends would draw too large a conclusion from my weeping and think their visits must be a terrible imposition, when the reality was that I could equally easily be crying about a baseball game. After I regained my composure, we were able to discuss various specifics, such as the use of the sponge around the sink and the definition of shouting versus talking, but I had the feeling that no amount of rational discussion could erase the gut impression that I must be terribly upset.

At the end of that same summer, Hurricane Katrina devastated New Orleans. Our friends were in a dilemma. They had been driving home when the hurricane hit, but now they turned around and came back to Vermont. Their house was intact, but the city was pretty much shut down. Ruth and I talked about the situation and agreed to invite them to stay with us for as long as they needed to.

When Ruth's mother heard about this plan, she was worried that the prolonged upheaval might be a risk.

"Why don't I give them my apartment?" she suggested. "I could just stay where I am."

"Where I am" was the nearby country house she shared with friends every summer. Ordinarily she would move back to her own apartment in the retirement community in the fall. This offer to abandon her own plans was characteristic. She was always helping people.

What I saw was that two other households would be disrupted in order to protect my health, and I immediately objected.

I was adamant that I was not going to live like a delicate hothouse flower for fear of what "might" happen. I suppose it sounded contradictory, since I had raised the question of stress reduction earlier in the summer. But now the situation was different. Our friends had a real crisis in their lives. Whatever might happen with my health was hypothetical. I knew what I would do if I didn't have MS: I would welcome them to stay with us. I wasn't going to act differently because of a speculative risk.

This insistence had an element of superstition. Or perhaps it could be called placebo management, if the real meaning of placebo is the power of the mind to affect the body. Living with MS felt like being in a perpetual game of chance, and people in such situations often make superstitious bargains with the universe. One of the bargains I had made was that, as long as I was healthy, I would not use the potential threat of MS as an excuse to get out of a responsibility.

My life included several jobs I would rather not have been doing, mostly related to family business and property. Those jobs were far more stressful than the logistics of sharing a house with friends could ever be. I often was tempted to say, "I'm worried about my health. I'm resigning my position."

But that temptation felt even riskier than the stress itself. I really felt as though using the potential for future disability as an excuse to avoid an unpleasant task would invite the universe to make me disabled in fact. Perhaps it was superstition. Or perhaps it was respectful caution about the power of Pavlovian conditioning. I did not want to offer myself rewards for being sick. I did not want to train myself to be even sicker.

If the MS ever did get worse, I would deal with what it meant. In the meantime, I put my illness in the same category as my sister's shorthand phrase for any unpredictable catastrophe, "getting hit by a bus." I would never have said to my family, "I might get hit by a bus, so I'm turning this tedious job over to someone else." It seemed equally silly to say, "I might get sicker someday, so I'm going to act sick now."

10

KICKS UNDER THE TABLE

Two weeks after Katrina uprooted our friends, I got news that would turn my own family on its head. My mother had suffered a severe hemorrhagic stroke. She had been rushed to a medical center in Montana, a hundred miles from her home.

Ruth and her mother and I were on vacation at a beach cottage when the call came. Since my siblings and I were not big phone talkers, having my brother track me down there was ominous even before he said a word. After telling me what had happened, he helped my mother with the phone, and she managed a hoarse, garbled hello.

I told her I loved her, and then Ruth and I booked the soonest flight we could get. We threw all our vacation things into bags and boxes and drove north to Boston, where Ruth's mother dropped us off at the airport before continuing on to Vermont with the dog and most of our stuff.

When Ruth and I arrived at the hospital, my mother was unconscious, and her survival looked doubtful. All of my siblings had gathered there from different parts of the country, and a nephew had come with his baby, the newest great-grandchild. For the moment family irritations were put aside, and we waited together, each seeking our chosen form of comfort, whether hugs or prayer or medical data.

Although the hospital staff did not commit to a prognosis, they clearly thought the most likely slope of the curve was downward. My mother had a pool of blood the size of a large plum in her frontal lobe. She might not die immediately, but it was likely she would not regain consciousness and would slip away over time.

A month earlier she had been with us in Vermont, the last stop on a circuit of visits in New England. At eighty-six, she still made trips across the country by herself to see relatives, and on this trip she also had organized a weekend gathering of old friends at a country inn in western Massachusetts. Her walking had slowed, and she had started to use wheelchair assistance in airports, but her mind still bubbled with ideas.

Seeing her off at the airport, I had waited outside the glass walls while she went through security. I had watched as she laboriously bent over in the wheelchair to remove her shoes, handed over all the odds and ends she carried in her pockets, and spread her limbs to be scanned, and I had wondered if this could be the last time she flew across the country. Now, keeping vigil in her hospital room, my siblings and I didn't know if she would even get out of the hospital.

The doctors didn't think she would die that night; her body was tough and was likely to hang on for a while.

They advised us to go to our motel and get some sleep. But they did not make any predictions about the likelihood of recovery. All they said was, "Anything could happen."

The next morning, I walked into the hospital room, and the first thing I saw was my brother, grinning from ear to ear. I looked past him, and there was our mother, propped up on pillows, being helped to eat a bowl of oatmeal. Her left arm and leg were extremely weak, and she would need many weeks in a rehab facility to learn new coping systems, but she had survived. Being old had been an asset. The brain shrinks with age, so her skull had more space for the pool of blood. In a younger brain, the pressure from the pool would more likely have been fatal.

It soon became clear that my mother's biggest loss was in her executive and decision-making capabilities. As she put it, "I've lost my 'do-it' button." For someone who had spent her life managing a business, organizing events, giving speeches, urging congressmen to act, and leading the charge to improve the world in her chosen arenas of combat, this was a major change in character. One of her greatest pleasures in life had been organizing a good party, and now she could barely organize a set of clothing to put on in the morning.

Curiously, although she needed to be nudged to make decisions, she had not lost her determination once she set her mind on something. Even without her do-it button, she was a star patient at the rehab center, diligently working at every exercise and coping skill the staff taught her. She spent hours with occupational therapists, being instructed to grasp a ball, to move the ball out to the side or lift it over her head, all with the goal of rewiring the connection from her brain to the movement of her left hand. The effort was tiring, but she stuck with it. It's a mystery of brain layout that she could lose her decision-making ability but retain her tenacity in pursuit of a goal, in this case the goal of regaining function and going home.

In a sense she was still the head of the family. She represented an unswerving integrity and moral authority that still held some sway over her kids' behavior. All of us had witnessed her battles to challenge deceptive marketing and dishonest record keeping in the cattle business, and probably most of us had had personal childhood experience with her ethical standards.

One occasion still vivid in my mind was when I was in about third grade and invited the twenty or so kids in our two-room school to my birthday party but did not invite one girl who was new to the school. During the party, my mother somehow discovered I had left someone out and immediately drove to the girl's house to fetch her. She also had a chat with the teachers, and the next day the formidable woman who taught the "upper graders" took me aside for a talking to.

The teacher didn't raise her voice or express anger. She just said, "I think you should know that after you handed out your party invitations last week, Robin went home from school crying."

Without her saying another word, I understood that what I had done was contemptible. My mother wanted me to recognize the hurtfulness of excluding people, and I think she intuited, correctly, that the message would sink in more thoroughly if it came from the schoolteacher.

Now, after her stroke, my mother's integrity was still rock solid, but her new passivity changed the nature of our family organism. No one quite dared to engage in an open fight right in front of her, but the covert battles became more intense and bitter. We were like children trading kicks out of sight under the dining room table while smiling innocently and pretending we were just eating our dinner.

My mother was perfectly aware that the kicks were happening, but she had lost the ability to take charge and tell us to knock it off. I think for the last few years of her life, she suffered a form of intractable pain, knowing that her family was falling apart and there was nothing she could do to stop it.

Others in the family might have said that there had always been animosity between certain siblings, but some lingering remnant of my childhood-hero worship of all of them had made me oblivious. Perhaps they were right. But for me, prior to my mother's stroke, the support and stability of the family had far outweighed its frustrations. After her stroke, this was less clear. Our communication had mostly shifted to email, and as the conflict intensified, signing on to email felt like reaching into a dark hollow where there might be something warm and fuzzy, but more likely there was a rattlesnake.

Some of our difficulties had long been apparent, even to me. For almost thirty years, the siblings had been trying to agree on a plan for the future of the ranch, parts of which had been owned by our family since the 1890s. Every attempt dribbled away in futility. Our shared compulsion to plan for every contingency meant we could debate issues to eternity and never settle anything.

A lot of people would have been glad to have the dilemma we faced. Our big problem was that we owned a beautiful ranch in a world where such expanses of unspoiled landscape were steadily being carved up into lucrative residential developments. Sometimes the reason for the carve-up was a financial crisis, but often the reason was the situation we faced, a generational transition to multiple descendants, no one of whom could afford to buy out all the others and maintain a viable business with single ownership. For our family, it was work together or bust.

The most perplexing feature of our impasse was that we didn't disagree about the goal. We all wanted the ranch to stay in the family. We just had six different ideas about how to accomplish this and, in some cases, a missionary certainty that our own idea was the only right one.

When my mother lost the ability to participate, a discussion that had been merely frustrating became acrimonious. As the youngest child, I often was the one who looked for a compromise, but trying to be a mediator was folly. I was part of the situation myself, and both sides resented it if I said anything favorable about the other side's point of view. For me, the result was a maddening amount of time wasted and a lot of insomnia.

My visits to the ranch, which used to be joyful, became a compound of joy and dread. I could feel myself detaching, in self-defense. The more I cared, the more painful the conflict became. The only recourse was not to care so much.

The landscape hadn't changed. I love New England, but every time I flew into Wyoming, I could feel my heart lift and spread itself into the generous expanse of open space. The western horizon is a wall of mountains, dark blue-green with conifers, rising over thirteen thousand feet. At the foothills, the precipitously steep forest gives way to gently sloping benches of grassland, their seeming flatness split by water-carved draws that widen as they fall away from the mountains until they merge into a broad valley of hay meadows.

The bottomland, irrigated, is vivid green. The surrounding hills are brown nine months of the year, their dry soil sparsely covered in bunchgrass, yucca, and sage. In company with the grazing cattle, the pastures are teeming with wildlife, from deer and elk to coyotes, sandhill cranes, and meadowlarks.

Even when the hills are green, the green is pale to a New England eye. Only in the creek bottoms do trees survive, scraggly cottonwoods and box elders. Everywhere the geologic bones of the landscape are laid out in clear view.

My nose never drips in Wyoming the way it does in a New England winter. The air is too dry. When rain does come, the fragrance of dry grass and sage saturates the senses. Like the vegetation, the houses are widely scattered. Our ranch is in a thickly settled area by Wyoming standards, and my mother's house is half a mile from her nearest neighbor.

When I was a child, there was a house within a quarter mile, occupied by one of the families on the adjacent ranch, but with mechanization the ranches have depopulated, and that house is gone. Our ranch employs half the number of people it did in the 1960s and produces more. This has been an evolution driven by economic survival. In today's economy, a ranch couldn't stay in business if it employed the number of people that was typical fifty years ago.

In concert with the depopulation of the ranches themselves, which used to be almost small villages, the central town has spawned a mushroom growth of mini-ranch

commuter subdivisions on what used to be hay meadows and pastures. One of these subdivisions grew up on
the wide meadow around our community clubhouse, the
old log building that housed dances, potluck suppers,
Halloween parties, and farm bureau meetings all through
my childhood. In a painfully symbolic coincidence, not too
many years after the subdivision replaced the hay meadow,
the community clubhouse burned down and has not been
rebuilt.

When I was growing up, I did not feel that our home
was in any way remote. "Remote" was my father's cousin
in Montana, whose ranch was forty miles from any settle-
ment bigger than a bar and gas station, and several miles
from a neighbor. Our house was only fourteen miles from
a substantial town, and ten of those miles were on pave-
ment. We were only four miles from the rural grade school
and the cluster of houses around it. We had neighbors up
and down the road, every half mile or so.

The schoolhouse sat at the hub of several gravel roads,
none of which had enough kids to justify a school bus, so
my mother took turns with the other parents on our road,
carpooling all the kids to the school. There, a bus from town
collected the high school kids and also dropped off the two
teachers for the grade school, saving them the ten-mile
drive. No one thought about "greenness" or "virtue" in this
sort of transportation economy. It was common sense. For
the most part, it has gone the way of the large ranch crews,
the community clubhouse, the municipal swimming pool,
and the small factories we would visit on school tours—
businesses that once produced local brands of sugar, flour,
potato chips, and ice cream; packed local meat; and bottled
Coca-Cola, all in a town of eleven thousand people.

Today, people have satellite TV and smartphones. Instead of going to a municipal pool, they build their own private swimming pools or join a health club. The buildings that were flour mills and creameries are now motels, banks, and shopping centers. Flour, sugar, and ice cream arrive on long-distance trucks for distribution to Safeway and Walmart. Production is more efficient, household income is higher, and people prefer the convenience of taking their own car whenever they go somewhere. The rural elementary school is closed, and the few remaining kids in our neighborhood go to the larger schools in town.

The family house that had been part of a lively neighborhood when we were children took on a different aspect when we needed people to help with my mother's care after her stroke. From the perspective of people who lived in town, the house was a long way out on what seemed like a very empty road, a road that in winter could be treacherous with whiteouts and snowdrifts. If a blizzard came, it wasn't a matter of hunkering down and staying home the way we would have when we were children. My mother depended on someone being there.

When the time came for my mother to move back to her house, my family was in a state of perpetual argument, so we argued about this decision too. What if she needed to go to the hospital? What if the power went out? There was a nice retirement community in town where she would be safer and have more company. The points in favor of town were reasonable, but my mother had her own view. She wanted to live on the ranch, in her own house.

She wasn't worried about the extra distance to the hospital, and she had less and less desire to interact with other people. The "company" at the retirement center would be more wearing than pleasant. What she really wanted was to sit quietly, to be read to, to watch a movie or an episode from her complete collection of *M*A*S*H*, to look out the window at her bird feeders, to nap. She liked the company of people she was close to, her family and a small number of longtime connections, but she wanted those people to do most of the talking and let her sit and listen.

For me, her passivity was a strange reversal. For most of my life, she had operated in a whirl of energy and enthusiasm that tired me out. She was a natural-born executive, happy to delegate, and eager to share her ideas with anyone who came in range. She didn't enjoy fun activities nearly as much as she enjoyed encouraging other people to enjoy fun activities. In our phone conversations, my half had usually been a periodic "Uh-huh," to let her know I was still there listening. When I did try to get more of the airtime, the effort to break in on her stream of talk had felt like a shout of insistence.

Now, instead of trying to squeeze in a few words here or there on a phone call, I had to chatter away like a radio announcer, filling the empty space. Sometimes a topic caught her interest, and she would talk, but often I found myself pausing to ask, "Are you still there?" to which she would answer "Yes," unless her hand had gotten tired, and the phone had slid away from her ear.

In the year she turned ninety, I asked her what she would like to do to celebrate. She said she would like a gathering at our family vacation place at the seaside in Massachusetts. I think she imagined all her children together there, as they had been for her eighty-fifth birthday, when we still maintained an illusion of amicability. Also, although she had very little stamina, she wanted her trip to include a stop in Maryland to visit one of my sisters who was undergoing chemotherapy for multiple myeloma and could not travel. The birthday trip was complicated and expensive to organize, and virtually every detail became a topic for argument among the siblings, the subject of dozens of contentious emails in the weeks leading up to her departure.

When it finally happened, the seaside gathering included only a small fraction of the family who had celebrated five years earlier, but for those few days my mother was very happy. She could see the ocean from her chair in the living room. In the daytime, we had a golf cart to take her to the beach. In the evening, she could rest in her chair, joining us in a card game or listening as we talked or played chamber music. On the last day, as I drove her on the first leg of her trip home, she started to weep and said, "I don't want to leave."

A few months later, when I visited her in Wyoming, she said she was going to die very soon. I asked her why she thought that, and at first she wouldn't say. Finally, she said she didn't want my sister who had cancer to die before she did. Even though we both knew many people who had been saved by treatment, she still thought of cancer as fatal. For her, no number of people on the plus side could overbalance the loss of my father.

It took a while to convince her that the chemotherapy really was working, and my sister really was in remission. Once she digested this fact, she decided she didn't need to be in such a hurry to die.

11

THE QUIET HOUSE

In the year after her ninetieth birthday, my mother began to need transfusions to keep her hemoglobin at adequate levels. She had a blood condition related to leukemia that caused her to produce abnormal white cells and platelets, and the doctors had put her on a chemotherapy that countered the abnormality but also depleted her red cells. She had very little stamina, but she was remarkably cheerful.

She also was losing weight. Throughout her widowed life, she had been very heavy, around two hundred pounds. She had talked about the need to lose weight and had made sporadic attempts to do so, but she had never succeeded because her energy and vigor found outlet in mental and social activity, not physical exertion. She liked to joke, "Why stand when you can sit? Why sit when you can lie down?" Her most characteristic posture was sitting in her command-central easy chair in our living room, with a table full of papers and a cup of tea at her elbow, handling business on the phone. Except for dancing, she didn't like to exert herself.

Now, without trying, she was losing weight. Part of her was pleased that she was finally showing progress in a life-long battle. But part of her probably knew the truth, that her loss of weight was a sign she was starting to die.

Step by step, she was moving in that direction. For years, she had been cajoled or bribed into daily sessions on a seated exercise machine, mostly by the promise that her caregiver would read aloud to her for as long as she kept her feet pushing the pedals. She also had made laps around the house with her walker. But the machine sessions and the laps were getting shorter and shorter, and then they stopped altogether, and then she began to rely on a wheel-chair most of the time.

In the autumn, a bad reaction to a transfusion put her in the hospital for a few days. From the hospital, she was released to a rehabilitation center to regain strength.

Her previous stay at the rehab center, after her stroke, had been a triumph of determination. She had thrown her-self into the therapy sessions and didn't mind the institu-tional environment. She had a goal and the possibility of reaching it: to walk, to feed herself, to regain some auton-omy, and to go home.

This time, she hated being there, and her only goal was to go home. She was no longer in the rehab program with the people who were going to recover and resume their lives. She was in the waiting program with the people who were never going to get better.

The facility was chronically understaffed, and the aides were necessarily focused on doing her basic physical care as swiftly as possible, bundling her on and off the toilet, into her chair, into her bed. They were pleasant enough, but always in a hurry and sometimes less than gentle. After the hospital stay, she was too weak to use her own legs to help with transfers, so the aides used lift straps to move her. The straps were quicker, probably safer, and certainly better for the aides' backs, but they had the feel of the equipment used to move pianos and large bags of grain.

When we talked to her doctor about discharge, he said we needed to have a conversation with her, to find out what kind of care she wanted so he would know what orders to write. I never saw this doctor in person. I only spoke to him on the phone. But his way of talking reminded me of the firm but gentle pressure one is supposed to apply to certain wounds.

A few years earlier, after my mother's stroke, I'd had a conversation with her about what she wanted. She had already signed an advanced directive saying that she didn't want to be resuscitated when her heart stopped. But then I asked her specifically, "If you have another episode like the stroke, where you're unconscious but breathing, do you want to be taken to the hospital?" She said yes, absolutely. She wasn't refusing medical care if she was alive. She just didn't want to be resuscitated.

This time, when my brother and I talked to her about what she wanted, she was equally clear. She wanted to go home. She did not ever want to go into the hospital again, for any reason. She did not want any more transfusions. She would continue the routine of pills she'd been taking, for her blood condition, but she did not want any new medical care whatsoever. She was willing to take Tylenol for the shoulder she had bruised falling out of bed in the rehab center and for the knee that had troubled her for fifty years, ever since a skiing accident.

Her doctor signed the discharge order, with care instructions reflecting her wishes. The red cells from her last transfusion would live about three months, until sometime in January. He couldn't predict how long she would live, but without transfusions, she would get steadily weaker.

She went home just before Thanksgiving. For the holiday, both of my brothers were planning to be away from Wyoming, visiting their own children, so Ruth and I flew west again to spend some time with her. We cooked a turkey dinner. We watched her favorite movie, *Murphy's Romance*, for about the fifth time in my case, and about the fiftieth in my mother's. I read books to her, and Ruth and I chatted with each other and with the caregivers. For the most part, my mother stayed quiet, listening. After the holiday, Ruth flew home, and I stayed on a while.

Among other things, I was struck by the quiet of her house. When I was a child, the house was never silent. Always, there were visitors—cattle buyers, foreign exchange students, vacationing cousins, and friends. The phone rang constantly, and conversations with my mother were rarely brief. The cook would be busy in the kitchen, and my mother usually had a secretary helping her with the ranch business. We had a Norwegian elkhound, famously fond of barking, and outdoors we had horses, sheep, and barn cats. The seven kids spent a lot of time reading, but we also played games and engaged in recreational argument. And always at the center was my mother, whirling through the household in a permanent state of having too little time for all the things she wanted to do.

Now the house was very still. My mother napped much of the time. Deer and wild turkeys wandered through the front yard. The only centers of frenetic activity were the bird feeders outside the living room window.

My mother's whole life had been charged with restless energy and shot through with grief. She'd battled for progressive change, in the cattle business, in the environmental movement, in alternative health. She'd resisted getting old, keeping her hair dyed and her attitude forward. She liked action and preferred the company of younger people. In recent years, I sometimes felt that she was fighting to keep herself alive in the hope of seeing her family heal itself. It was almost as if she were trying to interpose her own frail body as a shield between the siblings who would otherwise be tearing at each other with bare claws.

That winter, for the first time since I'd known her, she had stopped fighting. With no more trips to the beauty salon, her hair began to grow in white. Parts of her body were uncomfortable, but she continued to decline any painkiller stronger than Tylenol. She did not seem defeated or resigned. Her attitude was more like resolution. She had decided to let go, and although she was physically weak and needed help with the smallest of personal tasks, she seemed surprisingly happy.

My sisters and I took turns flying to Wyoming to spend time with her, and she loved every visit, but when it became clear she was finally failing, she was equally clear that she did not want all of us to convene in a group and keep a hovering vigil. She'd had quiet time with each of us, except the sister whose health still prevented travel, and I think she wanted to carry on with her life until it ended, rather than having someone clink a glass with a spoon to stop the party and call everyone's attention to her departure.

She died at the end of March, in the company of my next older sister, her namesake.

12

ONE LESS WORRY

The telephone lines to my farm were old and sometimes made a distracting buzz in the background of conversations. For me, the years of sibling conflict felt like those disintegrating phone lines. My home life was happy, but my immediate happiness was accompanied by a background buzz of distress about my family.

Three months after my mother's death, that distress got a whole lot worse. On a bright summer morning, I was served with a summons to appear in court in Wyoming.

Now that my mother was not there to see it, my oldest brother had filed a lawsuit against four of his younger siblings, including me. It seemed he thought the court would be a fast way to solve our business problems, or at least his part of them. With his eye on his own goals, he couldn't see that hauling us in front of a judge and putting forward unfounded accusations of malfeasance might make us mad. It was as if he thought a court battle was sort of like a hockey game, where players might trade punches to blow off steam but afterward could all go out to a bar together.

He also didn't realize how long it takes for anything to make its way through the courts.

If it had been a television drama and not my life, I might have found the litigation interesting. In fact, our case was so interesting that when it went to appeal to the Wyoming Supreme Court, it was chosen as the demonstration case to be argued in front of the annual convention of the state bar association. I had to buy new clothes to try to look formal and professional sitting in the front row of the convention hall with the justices up on the stage, the lawyers in front of them presenting arguments, and the audience behind us watching it all.

I can laugh now, sort of, because we won, but for years the litigation was agonizing and exhausting. I had to watch my sister—one of the most honest and least conniving people I know—in the witness box being questioned by an attorney who was trying to spring traps to make it look like she had done something wrong. My email inbox became an incessant barrage of communications about the case with lawyers and my siblings. Instead of writing fiction, I was helping to draft legal briefs, and I learned more about our court system than I had ever intended. Especially I learned the hazards of running a business on a handshake basis, as our family had done for decades, if somebody wanted to make trouble.

Even before my brother's lawsuits (which would multiply), our constant family arguments had accomplished nothing. They had been a waste of time and energy, a source of insomnia, and a barrier to progress in our shared business concerns. They probably had aggravated the frightening nightmares and delusions my mother had been suffering, which often involved threats to one of her grandchildren. In my own work life, I had not been able to focus my thoughts to make fruitful progress on another book.

But with litigation, we were not only wasting countless hours but also spending horrifying amounts of money, and the experience was shredding whatever was left of the personal affection between the one brother and the rest of us. In business we would continue to carry out obligations properly, but as family we had little desire to sit down for a nice dinner together.

There was one small piece of good news in this mess, however, and that was my health. As the arguments went on for year after year, I had lost sleep, stayed thin, inflicted my irritability on Ruth, and felt my tension migrate from one nagging sore place to another—back, neck, hip, ankle. Probably every hour of nighttime ceiling gazing was stiffening my arteries, weakening my memory, and lopping the youth-preserving telomeres off my chromosomes. And yet, through all of this, my MS symptoms had stayed dormant.

Much of the literature on MS had suggested that stress might increase the likelihood of a flare-up. Now, thanks to my family situation, I had just subjected myself to a multi-year test of this possibility. The result, in my case, seemed to be negative. Stress by itself had not caused my MS to relapse.

This did not mean stress was harmless. Conventional and alternative medical views agree that stress is bad for one's health. Unfortunately, even as human genius eliminates sources of stress from the past, such as losing one's child to diphtheria or one's wife in childbirth, we invent a multiplicity of smaller ways to raise our blood pressure, such as traffic jams, multitasking, and a niggling irritation whenever an electronic communication isn't answered within minutes. The modern merry-go-round keeps accelerating, and most of us choose to stay on it for fear we might miss something if we jump off.

I suppose it wasn't altogether rational to think, *Well, the last few years have been hellish, and I didn't have a relapse, so that's one worry off my list.* Like everything about my MS experiment, this observation was not scientific. I was a study group of one, and anything I experienced could be coincidence. Nevertheless, I did feel a sense of relief. It was bad enough to be stressed, without also worrying that the stress would cause something much worse.

So I had less cause for worry, but more cause for curiosity. If stress did not cause flare-ups, what did?

After my last flare-up, in 2004, the doctors had advised me to go on a medication that had limited effectiveness, caused negative side effects, and cost $1,400 a month. This advice felt like sirens going off and warning lights flashing. My condition must be terribly dangerous if such an expensive partial remedy was judged to be worth it. However, those same doctors couldn't say what had triggered the flare-up in the first place.

At the time, I had wondered about this question and made a list of potential culprits I could identify in my own experience. There were three of them: emotional stress, physical irritation of my spine, and a sandwich I had eaten.

When I made the list, stress had looked far and away like the front-runner. I was newly married, and the intensity of feeling made for bumps. The flare-up had begun within days after the death of my father-in-law. Emotions

had been powerful in both directions, positive and negative, and it seemed plausible that they were a factor.

But now, more than a decade later, I had a lot of evidence that emotional stress did not trigger flare-ups, so I
went back to take a look at my other two possibilities.

Physical irritation was on my list because, while Ruth's
father was in his final illness, I had tried to sleep on the
floor of the hospital waiting room and had spent much of
the night with my neck awkwardly kinked. One of my first
two flare-ups was also preceded by a strain on my neck,
from painting the ceiling of our porch. Could the strain
have started an inflammatory process that made a pathway for immune cells to attack the central nervous system?

In the books about MS, I could not remember any mention of physical irritation as a possible factor in the disease.
Also, in the years since 2004, I'd had many opportunities
to test what happened if I strained my neck, whether painting, doing carpentry, or trying to sleep on the floor of the
Denver airport on several occasions after my last-flight-of-
the-day to Wyoming had been missed or canceled. None of
these incidents had led to a flare-up.

The other candidate was a chicken salad sandwich.

While we were at the hospital with Ruth's father, someone in the group had gone to the delicatessen to bring back
sandwiches for lunch. I noticed that the filling of my sandwich was very creamy, but under the circumstances I did
not want to ask the person who had provided it whether it
had any milk in it. I just ate it and hoped the creaminess
came from mayonnaise rather than yogurt or sour cream.

In the nine years between 1995 and 2004, this was one
of the only occasions when I had eaten a food that might
have contained milk. At the time, I was not seriously

worried about it. Even if the chicken salad were laden with yogurt or sour cream, I doubted that a one-time serving of milk could precipitate a flare-up. If milk did contribute to flare-ups, I expected it was through a cumulative effect on immune function and not as a sudden reaction to a particular swallow of milk. It was not impossible that a few bites of yogurt could trigger an immune reaction. People with allergies to nuts or shellfish can react to a microscopic exposure. But I thought it was unlikely.

Unlike emotional stress and physical trauma, the creamy chicken salad has never been tested against subsequent experience. I can control my diet much more easily than I can control the sources of emotional stress, and my avoidance of milk has remained as absolute as I can make it. I suppose if I were truly dedicated to the pursuit of scientific knowledge, I would yield to the enticements of ice cream and butter cookies to see if eating them would precipitate a flare-up. I do wonder about it, but so far, my curiosity has not overcome my desire to stay healthy.

13

THE SLIPSTREAM

At the time my mother died, more than seventeen years had passed since my first episode of MS. Because I had been so lucky, I had had a kind of superstitious reluctance to talk much about the disease or my personal diet regimen. Partly I felt it could jinx me somehow, to make a big deal of it, especially when I had no scientifically meaningful data to back up my personal experience. Partly, I didn't want to proselytize.

Friends and family often passed along to me some new treatment idea that had popped up in the media—bee stings, vitamin D, intestinal parasites, among others—and I was glad to have the information, but I would quickly get irritated if the telling turned into urging. I assumed that others with MS would feel the same way if I started pushing my ideas onto them.

I didn't know anyone personally whose symptoms were severe. The people in my acquaintance who had MS were all doing reasonably well, some on medication, some not, some with dietary changes, some not. I had read or heard about people for whom the disease was incapacitating or even fatal, but I had never met them.

Then, about a month after my mother's death, Ruth and I traveled to Indiana University to attend the premiere of a film directed by Tom and Tracey's son, who was graduating in May. The film showing coincided with senior recitals in the music school, which also drew crowds of parents and friends to the campus.

In the course of the festivities surrounding these events, I met a lot of new people—the cinematographer, whose orange Mohawk matched his suit coat; the faculty adviser on the film, a geyser of enthusiasm about her students; various other family and friends, all of us gathered to nibble hors d'oeuvres and bubble with admiration about the film and the musical performances.

One of these acquaintances, the mother of a student who had worked on the film, attended all the events in a wheelchair. She was about my own age, and it turned out she had MS. Her son said that she could in fact walk, but she suffered debilitating fatigue, and the effort of walking even small distances would leave her exhausted. The wheelchair allowed her to save her energy and thus take part in the social activities.

After one of the music recitals, she and I chatted a bit, but not about MS. The focus was on the kids and their accomplishments. As we were talking about the recital, someone offered us plates of celebratory cake and ice cream. The cake was a homemade confection, slathered in creamy, buttery icing, delectable even to look at.

My response was automatic, a polite "No, thank you." My neighbor happily accepted and began eating the dessert.

As I watched her relishing the cake and ice cream while sitting in a wheelchair, I was cycling through emotions. Part of me, obviously, was thinking, *There but for fortune, . . .* and was grateful to be standing on my feet. It was well worth giving up cake and ice cream if the sacrifice kept me mobile and energetic. But another part of me felt like a sanctimonious health Puritan for coming to a party and then refraining from feasting. That part admired the spirit and cheerfulness with which my neighbor plunged into the festivities.

More than anything, though, I felt sadness and dismay, as if I were watching someone with emphysema light a cigarette, except that I did not have any scientific data underlying the dread I felt. Much as I was tempted to speak up, to tell her what my research had found and what my own results had been, I decided to stick to topics better suited to the occasion. I wasn't her doctor, and I thought her food choices were none of my business.

Later, I sounded out her son about whether she'd be interested in an exchange of information, and he said he would ask. I never heard from her, so I was glad I had kept my mouth shut at the party.

My mother would not have kept her mouth shut. She did not care if it was "not her business." If she saw a person doing something she considered foolish or damaging, she would urge them to change. If she had any idea she believed would benefit another person, she was determined to tell them about it. Her vocation in life was to seek out all the newest good ideas and convince other people to try them. If one of our ranch hands hurt his back, she would tell him about an alternative healer who was a "magician," and very likely she would also make the appointment, pay for it herself, and offer him a ride.

Religion she considered private, a matter to be left to the individual conscience, but on subjects she thought belonged in the public arena, such as the health of the planet and the health of the body, she was an unapologetic missionary, spreading the word about any knowledge she thought would help. She had little patience for hidebound institutions and conventional wisdom. One of her strongest expressions of scorn and frustration was the word "unimaginative," a description I heard her apply at one time or another to a remarkable array of individuals and institutions—travel agents, scientists, doctors, politicians, bureaucrats, government agencies, universities, hospitals, airport bookstores, and the customer service person with whom she had just finished talking on the phone.

I had spent a lot of my life fending off her ideas. I also had seen how, when our family went to a conference about issues in running a family business, my mother became a magnet to half the people in the room while her adult children remained silent observers on the fringe. Her enthusiasm tired me out, but for people outside her immediate family, she was a galvanizing force. At her memorial gatherings that summer, one in Boston, one in Wyoming, people I knew only slightly or not at all stood up to talk about how she had changed their lives.

For good or ill, I was not my mother. I certainly felt the same urge she would have felt, to try to rescue someone who might be harming herself. As I watched a woman eating ice cream while pinned to a wheelchair by fatigue, I kept thinking, *I have information that might make a difference in your life.* But I didn't like to intrude, so I remained the observer on the fringe, leaving her to her own path without any unwanted input from me.

I didn't forget about her, however. The threat that had been an abstraction was now present in my mind as an individual person whose life was completely changed by MS. I found it harder to put aside my annoyance that the conventional medical system had apparently not bothered to study something that seemed like an obvious target for research, the epidemiological connection between MS incidence and milk in the diet.

For myself personally, I was of two minds about the absence of data. If my diet was a placebo, it was working brilliantly, and there was no contrary information to undercut its effectiveness. As long as the medical community didn't bother to study my dietary regimen, I could go on happily believing that it worked.

But when I considered the possibility that my diet was not a placebo, that it might actually be making a difference, then I felt active rage at the possibility that half a million people in the US were being harmed by a simple lack of information.

For seventeen years I had treated my diet as purely my own concern. After meeting the woman at the film premiere, my attitude began to change. I was being pulled in the direction my mother would have taken, as if even now her energy was generating a race car slipstream and inviting me to tuck in behind and draft her. For her, it wasn't enough to think something. You had to do something.

In the months that followed, other incidents nudged me toward action. My clarinet had progressed enough that I was playing with a small community orchestra, and one evening at a rehearsal a fellow musician mentioned that her husband had MS. I had met him at orchestra events, and at first I thought he was another instance of a person only mildly affected, because he had no noticeable disability.

His wife said he was in fact doing very well, at present. As she talked more, the complications emerged. He exercised regularly and found it helpful but had to be careful not to overdo it, because of fatigue. He had had two hip replacements, largely due to damage from steroid treatments for severe relapses far in the past. He had tried interferon but reacted badly and was not currently taking any medication. She said it had been many years since he'd had a relapse bad enough to put him in the hospital.

In other words, he had had major consequences but had adapted, and life went on.

Around that same time, a friend sent me a link to a YouTube video of a doctor lecturing about how her own MS had benefited from a variation of the "Paleolithic" diet—lots of fish, meat, fruit and vegetables, very little milk or grain. The lecturer said that the diet had reversed her very significant disability, and she credited the nourishing properties of the foods in her diet for restoring the health of the cells in her brain.

In one regard, the video was an affirmation. Here was someone testifying that a change in diet had reversed the course of her MS, and one element of her diet was the same as mine, the absence of milk.

At the same time, I felt some skepticism about her emphasis on the need for enormous quantities of the vitamins and minerals in her chosen foods. From the start, she linked MS to other diseases of the nervous system, such as Parkinson's and Alzheimer's, and implied that they all resulted from a lack of crucial nutrients. Her analysis took no account of the actual mechanism of MS, the immune system attack on myelin, and the ways it is different from the mechanisms of Alzheimer's and Parkinson's.

The YouTube lecturer's dietary recommendations were daunting. Her visual displays included piles of seaweed and plates and plates of kale, all aimed at supplying a hefty enough dose of the positive nutrients. Only as a brief after-thought did she mention the possibility that the foods she had eliminated, the grains and milk, might have damaging effects.

I took the lecturer's word for it that her diet had worked for her. My question was, "Why?"

Was it really necessary to stuff down seaweed, meat, fish, and vegetables, and do without rice, bread, pasta, cheese, and ice cream? Was it really necessary to eat a pound of kale every day?

The question reminded me of a puzzle I had encoun-tered when I worked as a computer programmer. Back in the 1980s, I worked for a company that designed software for educational applications. I would write the code for an application and run it through a program called a compiler that translated what I had written into machine language instructions. One day, something in the code I had written caused the compiler to crash.

It was normal for the compiler to find problems in my code and return error messages telling me what I needed to fix. This was different. This was a bug in the compiler itself. The code I had written was perfectly legal, but it con-tained something that the compiler was unable to process without crashing.

My supervisor said I should send a bug report to the company that sold the compiler. However, the program code that was crashing the compiler was hundreds of lines long, and I hated to send off the whole pile of code with a note that "something in this undifferentiated mess is causing a problem." So I set about trying to isolate a smaller segment of code that could cause the compiler to crash.

At first I assumed the problem was the complexity of something I had written, and I expected my smaller segment to be fairly large. But as I carved away more and more code and zeroed in on the part the compiler couldn't handle, it proved to be far simpler than I anticipated. By the time I was done, I was able to write a legal sequence of just six lines of code that would cause the compiler to crash, and that was the sequence I put in my bug report.

A computer is much simpler than a mammal, and simpler to debug. Still, MS is a specific malfunction in the immune system, and it seemed possible that it might have a specific cause. Looking at the YouTube lecturer's diet, I wondered if the success she attributed to all the good things she had added to her diet might instead be the result of eliminating some particular bad thing. I wanted to see a research study that separated her diet into components and tested if there was some simple six-line piece of it that was the crucial bit.

In the winter, another piece of data added itself to my collection. Our dog Lark started losing pigment in the skin of her lips and nose. Over a period of weeks, skin that had been black developed irregular patches of pink, which grew progressively larger.

When the vet examined her, he said it was probably an autoimmune reaction. Her immune system was attacking her own skin pigment. We asked what caused it, and he said the cause wasn't known. We asked if there was a cure, and he said no. We could try supplements of vitamin E and zinc, which promote skin health in a general way, but Lark's dog food had plenty of vitamins, and the problem was not the result of a deficiency.

Then he pointed at a pink patch on one side of her nose and said if it spread to the other side, we should bring her back for another exam.

My reaction to his information was the same as my reaction to MS seventeen years earlier. This problem had to have a cause. Our lack of knowledge made it look like it came out of thin air, but something was causing it.

We looked at Lark's environment and came up with two potential culprits. One was her food. The problem affected her mouth. Maybe she was reacting to something in her food. The flaw in this possibility was that she'd been eating the same dog food long before she had the problem.

The more likely possibility was a hard nylon ring I had bought her as a chew toy. She loved the ring and chewed it constantly. The new ring looked similar to previous toys that had caused no problem, but this toy was the only identifiable factor in her environment that was completely new.

Figuring the changes could do no harm, we switched to a different formula of her brand of dog food, and we took away the new nylon ring.

Within days of these changes, the pink patches stopped spreading and began to retreat. Over the next couple of months, we watched the slow creep of black pigment, restoring itself to health. When she first went to the vet, she had lost pigment all the way around the outside of her mouth and up onto her nose. Three months later, she still lacked some pigment inside her mouth, but on her lips and muzzle, the black had returned to all but one tiny spot below her left nostril.

For me, watching Lark's skin restore itself felt like watching a visible representation of the hidden process that must happen when an MS flare-up ends, and the myelin in the central nervous system starts to heal itself. Bit by tiny bit, her body fixed the damage and returned to normal.

What couldn't be known, of course, was whether it was all a coincidence. Perhaps the autoimmune process was about to halt on its own when we decided to change her food and take away her toy. Like me, my dog was a sample size of one, and hence statistically meaningless.

If my priority had been data, I could have tried feeding her the old dog food or giving her the nylon ring back, to test if her pigment would get destroyed again. But my curiosity had limits. As long as the remedy kept working, I would stick with it.

The one certainty was that it was not a placebo. It may have been a coincidence, but it was not a placebo, because Lark did not know that what we did was intended to be a remedy. All she knew was that she now had a beef shinbone instead of a nylon ring to chew on.

14

CLIMATE, COWS, AND THE COMMON COLD

As events kept pushing me in the direction of writing an account of my experiment, I realized there was a very large gap in my knowledge. My experiment had been based on the data available in 1995, which was mostly epidemiological. In the decades since then, the research tools and knowledge had expanded dramatically, especially at the microscopic level of T cells, viruses, genes, proteins, and immunological regulatory mechanisms. The disease is still a medical whodunit, with no definite answers about the cause or a cure, but we have a lot more clues to study.

For years, my strategy had been to think about MS as little as possible. Now I became curious. What had all that new research discovered? Had it turned up new information that either supported or debunked my ideas?

Starting with the obvious, I searched public medical websites for scientific studies relating to milk and MS. An encyclopedia of medical research papers was now accessible online, at least in abstract form and often in their entirety. Had any researchers studied the effect of milk in the diet of MS patients?

The answer was no, or none I could find.

What I did find were two epidemiological studies that described the correlation between milk consumption and MS incidence at the population level. One of these studies was the one I already knew about, from France in the 1990s. The other had been done even earlier, in Germany in the early 1970s. But apparently, in the forty-odd years since the correlation was observed, no one had tested what happened if MS patients eliminated milk from their diet.

When I widened my search to diet in general, a few studies did turn up, usually relating to fat. One of the most interesting had examined whether dietary supplements of beneficial unsaturated fatty acids made any difference in MS. The result of that study was negative. Eating more of the "good" fats made no difference.

Having failed to find any medical data to prove definitively that my regimen was a placebo, I looked for research to explain why it might work. Along the way, I mentioned my project to my brother-in-law John, the cancer researcher, who promptly sent me recent journal articles that he thought were groundbreaking.

His own research studied T cells in connection to cancer treatments, but the articles he sent discussed T cells in connection to both cancer and MS. The articles reported on a property of T cells that may be the key to their role in MS: their susceptibility to cross-reactions with proteins other than the protein that was their original target.

T cells are the current prime suspect in the MS mystery. Normally, they are the good guys, the immune system cops who run around ridding the body of pathogenic viruses. In a person with MS, however, the T cells apparently decide that a protein in the body's own myelin is marking a pathogen and they set about attacking it.

As I delved into the materials John had sent, he became my research buddy at the other end of the phone line. I had a multitude of questions, and he loved to talk about immunology, so our conversations could go on a long time.

"What's an epitope?" I would ask.

"It's a little piece of protein the T cell uses to recognize a virus," he would say, and then patiently explain more details. The essence was that when a T cell met a new virus, it would identify the segment of protein and file it away for future reference so that it could quickly respond if that same virus showed up again.

"So the cross-reaction is when that T cell meets some other protein with the same segment and reacts as if it's a virus?" I asked.

"Exactly!" he said. "And what's so exciting in this new research is that it seems to be a really short piece of protein that is the crucial identifier. Much shorter than we used to think."

He was nearly breathless with enthusiasm about this breakthrough. In the case of MS, the researchers had shown two key points: myelin-reactive T cells taken from MS patients would cross-react with proteins from other sources, and only a very small and clearly defined matching segment was needed to trigger the cross-reaction. So the net was tightening.

If cross-reactions really were the mechanism for MS, the key question still to be answered was what real-world protein or proteins were triggering flare-ups. The first candidates I needed to investigate were the proteins in milk itself.

At least one autoimmune disease, celiac disease, is known to be a T-cell cross-reaction between a protein in grains like wheat and a protein in the digestive tract. However, MS is very different from celiac disease, and the intermittent nature of MS flare-ups made it unlikely that the triggering protein was a permanent component of milk. To be more certain of this, I spent considerable time with an internet database of proteins and some online analytic programs, comparing sequences in milk proteins with the known epitopes in myelin proteins. No smoking guns appeared; I found no matching segments.

So then I wondered if milk has elements that are only variably present, such as contaminants from manure or feed, or pathogenic organisms from the cattle themselves. Or could milk consumption change body chemistry in a way that facilitates the action of some other external factor?

For a long time, scientists have thought there may be a virus at the root of MS. However, despite extensive research efforts, no one has found a virus that infects the central nervous system during an MS flare-up. The new research on cross-reactions suggests that the role of the virus may be indirect. Rather than infecting nerve cells that then get destroyed by the immune system, the virus might give rise to cross-reacting T cells that also attack myelin.

Different researchers have proposed different ways these T cells might start to proliferate and attack myelin. One possibility is a re-exposure to the original virus.

Another possibility is that a weakening in the blood-brain barrier allows the T cells into the central nervous system where the myelin protein itself causes them to proliferate. (Ordinarily, the blood-brain barrier keeps T cells from passing from the blood into the spinal fluid, but inflammation can cause the barrier to become more permeable.)

A third possibility is that both elements are involved. In other words, a re-exposure to the original virus causes the cross-reacting T cells to proliferate at the same time that some other inflammatory factor weakens the blood-brain barrier and allows those T cells to pass into the central nervous system.

To find ways these possible mechanisms might be linked to milk, I pulled back to the wide view to look at patterns in milk production and consumption.

One feature of milk production that piqued my interest was silage, which is fermented vegetable material stored in airtight silos or plastic bags. MS is a cool climate disease, rare in the tropics, and silage is commonly fed to dairy cattle in cool climates but rarely fed to cattle in the tropics. Also, silage is laden with microorganisms, both the anaerobic fermentation bacteria that are part of the process of making it and the occasional contaminating organism, such as clostridium. Could bacteria, or the spores from bacteria, be present in milk, and could they change the composition of the gut flora in people who drink milk?

Like silage, the human gut is an anaerobic environment. Could a proliferation of unusual microorganisms in the gut be a source of inflammation that weakened the blood-brain barrier and allowed myelin-reactive T cells into the central nervous system?

While poking around on this topic, I ran across a study from Japan on the topic of gut flora and MS. This study found that the profile of gut organisms in people with MS was different from the profile of gut organisms in controls without MS. The authors of the study pointed to an increasing incidence of MS in Japan and hypothesized that the increase was linked to the Westernization of the Japanese diet. They did not single out a specific food, but the central finding of their paper, that the gut flora in MS patients was different from the flora in healthy people, supported the idea that something about the diet was a factor in MS.

I kept digging on this subject of Japan and especially on the topic of its increasing incidence of MS. In 1995, when I was first looking at the epidemiology of MS, Asia was the big exception to the pattern of MS being a disease of high latitudes and cool climates. Japan and much of China are cool climate countries, and yet they had a low incidence of MS at that time. They also drank very little milk.

My first question was whether the "Westernization" of the Japanese diet included an increase in milk consumption. I searched for data on dairy production and consumption in Japan and found that the answer was yes. Per capita milk consumption had more than doubled between the 1960s and 2012, although it was still considerably lower than in the US and northern Europe.

However, the article on dairy production in Japan contained another tidbit I found interesting. Along with the increase in milk consumption, there had been a dramatic change in the nature of Japanese milk production. In the early 1960s, the average size of a dairy "herd" in Japan was less than three cows. In 2012, the average herd size was seventy-two cows. In other words, the cattle that once were scattered in twos and threes among tiny farms all over the country had been concentrated into more industrial-scale modern dairies.

Historically, the increasing prevalence of MS has paralleled the rise in industrialization and urbanization of human society. And as populations grow more concentrated and interconnected, viruses have a field day, reveling in the abundance of hosts and the ease of transmission from one host to another and one population to another. If MS is in fact related to some common, nonlethal virus, could that virus have a bovine equivalent that was traveling in milk and re-exposing people to the relevant viral protein?

For some reason, I found myself thinking about calf scours, which had been a constant worry during calving season on my farm. Scours is an infectious disease that strikes newborn calves as they begin suckling milk. The calf develops severe watery diarrhea and will rapidly die of dehydration if not treated. It mostly affects calves kept in the close confinement of a dairy barn, but I had encountered a few cases in my pastured beef cattle, and I kept a close eye on the newborns. They could go downhill very fast if I didn't spot the symptoms.

I knew the treatment for scours was electrolytes and sometimes antibiotics, but I did not know what organism caused the disease. Now I looked it up.

The bacterial type of scours could be caused by a variety of bacteria, but the viral type was commonly caused by two specific viruses, a reovirus and a coronavirus. I located the two bovine viruses in the protein database I had been using and began comparing the amino acid sequences in the viral proteins with the sequences in myelin.

Bingo.

A protein in the bovine coronavirus had a sequence matching the sequence in a myelin epitope.

Now I began studying up on the coronavirus. What were its properties? Did it have a human equivalent?

Again the answers were interesting. The bovine coronavirus does have a human equivalent, called OC43. It is one of the viruses that causes the common cold. (It should be noted that these coronaviruses are unrelated to the COVID-19 virus responsible for the deadly pandemic.)

The OC43 virus actually has two pathways to infection, a respiratory pathway and an enteric (digestive tract) pathway. In humans, the respiratory infection is the one that people usually experience. In cattle, both types of infection are common, but the pattern of infection is distinct. The respiratory infection is common in adult cows; the enteric infection is common in calves. Only the enteric infection causes big problems, so that is the infection that gets identified and treated.

Three other properties of the coronavirus caught my attention. First, in the course of a respiratory infection, the virus can sometimes find its way into the central nervous system.

Second, the coronavirus is sensitive to heat. It proliferates in cool environments and dies out in hot ones. So it fits the climate pattern in the distribution of MS.

Third, the adult cows with a respiratory virus infection shed the virus into their milk. They also secrete antibodies (immunoglobulins) to the virus into their milk.

It turns out that the coronavirus may be as common in modern dairies as the common cold is in people. In the United States, calf scours kills more calves than all other calfhood diseases combined. In Great Britain, a veterinary study tested the milk in bulk tanks on dairies around the country and found measurable antibodies to the coronavirus in every dairy they tested.

What this means is that people drinking the milk from these modern dairies in cool climates are ingesting both the virus and the bovine antibodies to the virus. The virus itself would not be alive in the milk. Pasteurization would kill it. But could the killed virus still prompt an immune response, in the same way that a killed virus in an oral vaccine can prompt an immune response? Or could the bovine antibodies interact with the human immune system in some way?

Having looked at the agricultural angle, I went back to the medical databases. Had anyone studied the OC43 virus in connection to MS?

Once again, the answer was yes. A research team in Quebec had published papers describing experiments that demonstrated a T-cell cross-reaction between a protein in myelin and a protein in the human coronavirus OC43. This research was only concerned with the human virus, but the bovine virus contained the same segment of protein that was involved in the T-cell cross-reaction. So it was at least theoretically possible that the bovine virus could trigger the cross-reaction, if there was a pathway by which human T cells could be exposed to it.

I now had information supporting two completely different potential explanations for a link between milk and MS. The Japanese study on gut flora pointed at a pathway involving inflammation and a weakening of the blood-brain barrier. The data from the dairy industry and the Quebec studies pointed at a pathway more directly involving a virus and the T cells themselves.

At this point, I had about reached the end of what a curious layperson could discover by poking around in the published research of scientists. None of what I had found proved anything, of course. The connections I had found could easily be a long series of coincidences that I happened to notice because I was looking at data from a particular angle that interested me.

If I wanted reasons for skepticism, I could find them easily. The reason that lived with me always was the unpredictable character of the disease itself. On one day I would find a research paper that seemed promising. On another day I would converse with an acquaintance with MS who had not had an acute flare-up in the last fifteen years, even though he took no medication and had not changed his diet. I never forgot that my own good results could be chance, and I never forgot that my own disease could change course at any time.

On the whole, I hoped that our medical system would someday investigate the same connections I was looking at. But a little piece of me was relieved that they hadn't, because, along with the possibility that a study might identify a clear link between milk and MS, there was also the possibility that a study might prove that avoiding milk had no effect whatsoever, and that I had been doing without cheesecake, nachos, and butter cookies for no reason at all.

15

DR15

Throughout my experiment, I had been a solitary lab rat. Now the question occurred to me, "How good a test subject was I? Was I a fairly typical MS patient, or was I an oddity?"

In other areas of my life, I didn't feel that I was an oddity, although people looking from the outside sometimes thought otherwise. One of my high school friends once said she was envious that after getting a fine college education I could be content living on a farm, doing odds and ends, renovating a house, and writing a few novels with a modest audience, rather than pursuing a high-level career of some kind.

Much of the world might have thought my being gay would make me feel I didn't fit, but here I was saved by my family, and particularly my mother.

At one point, early in my first sustained relationship and before I had come out publicly, my partner and I were snuggled together in one of the two beds in my childhood bedroom when we heard my mother coming up the stairs that led to the room. Leaping out of the bed, I snatched my nightgown and bolted across the room toward the other bed.

I made it halfway. When my mother opened the door, I was standing in the middle of the room, naked, covering my front with the nightgown, trying to pretend I had just started getting dressed for the day.

She didn't say anything in particular at that moment, maybe "Good morning," before pursuing whatever topic had led her to come up to my room in the first place. But not long after that, she asked me if I would like to join her at a conference on "love" that was happening at a college in Montana, a couple of hours from our house. In the car on the way home from that conference, she asked me, very delicately, "Are you having a woman relationship?"

I said, "Yes," and that was that; I was out.

I don't remember exactly how I told my various siblings, but their reaction was characteristic. "Oh, OK." And a shrug. And no measurable change in how they acted toward me. With that kind of solid ground under my feet, there wasn't much the wider world could do to make me feel odd.

As far as how I compared to the people I knew with MS, I couldn't see any pattern of either similarity or difference. It seemed to me they were about as varied as any random sample of the people I knew. Only one of them was gay. Another had played in the orchestra with me. A couple were physicians. One was my cousin. None of them were part of my closest circle of friends.

One of the more memorable occasions for comparisons happened at the wedding of my youngest niece. When Ruth and I sat down for dinner at our assigned table, we saw no one else we knew. However, one gentleman had arrived on a mobility scooter, which led to him explaining that he had MS. That announcement prompted a more general conversation about MS, in which it turned out that everyone at the table had some connection to the disease. One couple's son had just been diagnosed. Another woman had it herself and was recommending a special type of mushrooms as a treatment. Beyond acknowledging that I had MS, I didn't talk a lot about my situation, partly because several other people seemed very eager to talk. I still don't know if my niece had intentionally put us all at the same table with the idea that we would then have something to talk about, or whether it was pure coincidence. But as a sample of people with MS, it was as varied as the people I already knew.

The real question wasn't whether I and other people with MS shared a taste in music or a fondness for bagels. The question I wanted to know about was whether we shared any underlying physiology. Suppose my diet really had made a physical difference. Was it likely to make a difference for anyone else?

Along with environmental factors, MS is thought to have a genetic component, a predisposition that makes some people more likely to be affected by the disease. The T-cell response to proteins is governed by a set of genes known as the human leukocyte antigen (HLA) complex.

T cells do not look at the whole protein to identify it. They look at just a small segment. And different T cells may look at different small segments of the same protein.

If a protein is like a face that T cells learn to recognize, then one T cell may use the nose or the eyebrow to make the identification while another uses the chin or the ear. The HLA types of the T cell determine which segments of a protein that T cell will look at and recognize.

If a T-cell cross-reaction is indeed at the root of MS, then two things must be true. First, the myelin protein must have a segment that matches a segment in the external triggering protein. Second, the T cells must belong to an HLA type that can recognize that particular matching segment. Certain HLA types are known to be associated with a high incidence of MS, and this is one reason scientists suspect that a T-cell cross-reaction is part of the mechanism leading to MS. The configuration of HLA types that is most common in MS patients is known by a shorthand designation, "DR15."

Scientists do not yet know if there is a single factor that can be connected to all cases of MS, or if there are a number of different "varieties" of MS, possibly correlating to specific HLA types responding to different external factors. If there are many varieties, then a remedy that works for one person might be ineffective for another.

It is now possible to identify a person's HLA types, in the same way that a person's blood type can be identified. However, in contrast to the very limited number of blood types, there are hundreds of different HLA types. Some are quite common. Others are extremely rare. If I wanted to know if I was a good lab rat, genetically representative of a large number of MS patients, or a poor lab rat, a genetic rarity whose experience would not be relevant to anyone else, then I needed to find out my HLA types.

This turned out to be more complicated than I anticipated.

I was prepared to pay for the tests myself, but a willingness to pay was not the only issue. One cannot just walk into a lab, slap down one's credit card, and say, "I would like these three tests, please." I needed a physician to order the tests.

I scheduled an appointment with my primary care doctor to discuss the question. Dr. Clement had retired, and my new doctor at the clinic was a woman with many wonderful qualities, not the least of which was that she was much younger than I, so I could hope she would be practicing for many years. Dr. Bright was also upbeat, open minded, easy to talk to, and thorough.

At the appointment, I explained that I wanted the test purely for my own research, to satisfy my curiosity, and that I was prepared to pay the cost, if it was not exorbitant. Dr. Bright said she would be glad to order the tests but would have to figure out what diagnostic code she could use to order them. No treatments for MS depend on HLA type, so there was no code that obviously fit the situation.

She said the most common reason for HLA tests was for organ and tissue transplants, but they were sometimes ordered in cases of inflammatory arthritis. Did I happen to have any chronic joint pain? I said I'd occasionally had an aching joint, usually when I'd been cutting brush or digging postholes, but I had no pain that didn't eventually go away. She said my type of aching joint would be osteoarthritis, if it were any kind, and would not be a reason for an HLA test.

Dr. Bright seemed more bothered than I was that I might have to pay the cost myself. As she pointed out, if

I had been on MS medications since 2004, my insurance company would already have paid something like a quarter of a million dollars for my care. It seemed outrageous to her that I should have to pay the few hundred now for the HLA test. I said I could live with it, because I really wanted the information. On the whole, given a choice between paying for the test myself or suffering from an excruciatingly painful disease that would justify insurance coverage, I preferred to pay for the test.

Eventually, Dr. Bright figured out a category that would allow the test to be ordered. To find out what it would cost me, I would have to contact the lab at the medical center that would do the test.

As usually happened whenever I sought information about the cost of medical care, the people I talked to were pleasant and did their best to be helpful, but they were operating in a Byzantine payment system in which no one really knows what anything costs, because the price depends on who is paying and what deal they have negotiated with whom. I was directed from the lab to another administrative office in the hospital, and then from that office to a central office in another city, and then back to yet another office at the hospital where I met an answering machine that directed me to leave a message and they would get back to me.

The "getting back to me" required a follow-up phone call, and when I finally did get a cost estimate, it was prefaced by a lengthy disclaimer explaining that the complete circumstances could not be known ahead of time, and thus the actual cost might be quite different from the estimate. This final statement was accurate.

But in the end, my blood was drawn, the tests were done, and the cost, although higher than the estimate, was not a different order of magnitude.

The final step in the process was getting the lab results from the clinic to me, the patient. In the internet age, one would think the clinic could simply email the results to me. But because of the privacy requirements of HIPAA, they instead had a system that involved a "patient portal," which required a username and password to access. I never received any information directly by email. Instead, I received an email that said there was a message waiting for me inside the portal.

This layer of security applies even to general public announcements. Rather than sending me an email that says, "We are offering drop-in flu vaccinations next Tuesday," they send an email directing me to the portal. So I dig into my file of passwords to remember how to get into the portal, log into the portal, and navigate my way to the message section. I open the newest message, and lo and behold, I learn that the clinic will be offering drop-in flu vaccinations on Tuesday.

In the case of my HLA test results, the clinic attempted to convey the results by way of the portal. But for some reason the format in which they had received the results was not compatible with the system of posting lab results on the portal. So they sent me a message and said they would have to give me a paper copy. I said that would be just dandy, and I would pick it up the next time I was in town.

When I arrived at the clinic, the receptionist handed me a sealed envelope. I went out to my car before opening it. Contemplating the envelope, I felt a little of the nervous anticipation I had felt back when I was opening letters from colleges announcing acceptance or rejection.

The print was faint and fuzzy, but the result was not. My HLA types included the two alleles DR15:01 and DQ06:02, often lumped together and referred to as simply DR15, which were the types most commonly associated with MS. So I was not an outlier. Genetically, I sat right in the fat part of the curve of MS distribution, and if anything in my experience turned out to have any significance, it might well have significance for a lot of people.

16

SHY PERSON

For years, I had put aside my brother's suggestion that I write about multiple sclerosis, because I didn't want to sit at my desk every day and think about having the disease. In general, I tried to think about MS as little as possible. I would tell myself, *Maybe someday I'll write about it, but I'll wait until I've stayed healthy for a few more years . . .*

I think it scared me to write about how lucky I had been. My upbringing had infused me with New England caution, which greets good news with a reflexive "We'll pay for it later," and I felt a superstitious worry that talking too much about my good luck might cause it to change.

Then, as I began meeting more people who were seriously affected by MS, I found myself thinking a lot about my mother.

In the last years of her life, my siblings and I were so preoccupied with her need for care it was hard to remember the person who once cared for us. Instead of being a fountain of ideas about helping others, she had become the one who needed help. Instead of fending off her enthusiasm, we had to cajole her to take an interest in the world. As I grew accustomed to this passive, retiring personality, I somewhat lost sight of the dynamic person she had been for the eighty years prior.

After she died, that other person came charging back into my memory, vivid and full of vigor. The banner she was carrying said, "Get up and do something. Or stay sitting down and do something. But do something."

The corollary to her message was that no one is fearless, unless the person has disconnected from reality. Everyone encounters good reasons to be frightened, from piano recitals and job interviews to military deployments and mortal illnesses. The question is how to handle the fear. Do I let it govern me? Or do I nod good morning, offer it the passenger seat, and suggest it fasten its seat belt before the two of us set off together?

Now, along with the sparrow of MS, I had my mother perched on my shoulder, telling me to stop being superstitious and do something useful with my experience.

Around this same time, I happened to talk with a close friend, who had just returned from a vacation in the Caribbean.

"How was the trip?" I asked, and there was a pause.

Then she replied that her feelings were mixed. The Caribbean was lovely, but while she was there, she had gotten word that one of her oldest friends, someone she'd known since college, had died rather suddenly from complications of MS.

"I'm so sorry," I said. "That's really sad."

Knowing I had an interest in the disease, she told me more about what had happened. "My friend did well for years after the diagnosis," she said. "But then last winter she started going downhill very quickly and became quite incapacitated. She got so laid up, she ended up getting pneumonia."

I didn't say anything, but I could feel a little shot of fear, being reminded that my own disease could "go bad" at any time.

"Quite a while ago, I told her about your idea about milk," my friend said, "but she was doing the chemotherapy her doctors had recommended, and she wasn't interested in lifestyle changes."

Now what I felt was anger, thinking about the potentially helpful information that was not even on the radar screen of our medical establishment.

Would the friend have reacted differently if the suggestion about diet had come from a doctor rather than a random stranger with no medical training? Possibly not. Our national statistics on obesity, smoking, and lack of exercise indicate that legions of people pay no attention to the lifestyle recommendations of their doctors. But some people do pay attention. At least if patients are given the information, it is their own choice to ignore it. If patients never get the information in the first place, then the system has preemptively made their choice for them.

My mother would never have accepted this state of affairs. If she had an idea she thought was useful, she would not have been content to let the experts take their own sweet time investigating it. She would not have been willing to apply her good idea to her own life and let others make their own choices. She would have been buttonholing politicians and hammering on the doors of the people with "credentials," demanding that they listen to her and do something. Many of her ideas went nowhere, and some of them were downright nutty. But sometimes she got hold of a good idea, and her tenacity made a difference.

As measured by public name recognition, her effect was felt mostly in the cattle business and in her own Wyoming community, but she accomplished other things that don't have her name on them in any public way. In the personal arena, she left behind a lot of younger people who were inspired by her openness to new ideas and her "go for it" attitude. In the political arena, her badgering of people in power helped make at least one good law.

Sorting through her papers after her death, my sisters came upon a letter from the Jimmy Carter White House. The letter thanked my mother for her contribution to the passage of a bill requiring the reclamation of land that had been strip-mined for coal and invited her to a reception at the White House to celebrate the new law.

My family knew that after my mother turned management of the ranch over to her sons, she had spent years on the warpath about environmental issues, including nuclear power and especially coal strip-mining, which was ravaging the landscape in a nearby part of Wyoming. She had been connected to a number of regional environmental groups, and, being a natural networker, she was personally acquainted with many activists. It was pleasing to learn that all her conversations and conferences, all her racing about, had had a real-world effect.

Our most recent discovery about her life is a minor, but to us delightful, curiosity: her first Xerox copier is in the Smithsonian Museum. We know this only because

Ed, the man who used to repair her copiers, happened to take a vacation in Washington DC. When he visited the Smithsonian, he saw a machine on display as an example of the first generation of copiers and thought, "Boy, that sure looks like Sal's old machine."

Unable to contain his curiosity, he crawled under the machine, found the plate with the serial number, and wrote it down. When he got home to Wyoming, he dug into his records to find the serial number of my mother's Xerox. The numbers matched. The machine in the museum was hers.

My mother had acquired a Xerox machine almost the first moment they became available. For her it was a tool of propagation. Whenever she found new and interesting ideas in print, she made photocopies and sent them to everybody she thought might be interested. Decades before the internet, she had found a small way for a private citizen to try to make something "go viral."

Although she was quick to try new things, when she found a tool that worked, she liked to hold on to it. Ed was intimately familiar with her first Xerox machine because she had kept it for years and years, scorning all the newer models with more bells and whistles and begging him to find replacement parts to keep the old one running. Through most of a lifetime in Wyoming, she retained her New England reluctance to discard anything with a scrap of usefulness left in it. Our family speculated that her machine might have made its way to the Smithsonian because she had kept it in service long after all the other machines from that first generation of copiers had been junked.

She also held on to ties of affection. Her acquaintance with Ed had started with his job as a technician, but over the years he and his wife and kids would become among her closest friends, and they would continue to be her friends until the day she died, long after Ed had retired from maintaining her copier.

My mother was the sort of person who would stand up and give speeches to an industry of mostly conservative male ranchers, telling them the times are changing and they'd better wake up. She was someone who would invite her still-closeted daughter to join her at a conference about love and then use it as an entry to ask about my girlfriend, thereby relieving me of the anxiety about how and when to come out to her. She was someone who would pester congressmen about strip-mining and end up with an invitation to the White House.

Much as I admire her, I can't operate the way she did. I haven't a shred of her charisma or executive ability. At a party, I'm one of the listeners who feed laughter and setup lines to the entertainers in the crowd. I have very few beliefs for which I can't see a persuasive counterargument, and I treat advertising as a warning: the more a product is advertised, the greater the probability that it is either bad for you, overpriced, or unnecessary, and possibly all three. The net result is that I will never be a successful promoter. I may write a letter to my congressman, but I will never march into his office to demand that he listen to me.

When I heard my mother's voice in my head urging me to "do something" about MS, it was never an option to do what she would have done. Instead, I did what a shy person does. I sat down at my desk, in solitude, and started writing.

I would spend a great many hours studying a disease I really didn't want to think about. I would spend a great many more hours remembering a person I was glad to think about, my mother. And in thinking about those two things, I would come to wonder if the approach to life I absorbed from the one might possibly have saved me from the other.

ACKNOWLEDGMENTS

I owe boundless gratitude to the many people who have helped me in the shaping of this book.

First and foremost I want to thank my sister Cherry and my brother-in-law John Wunderlich. Starting long before this book was even thought of, John has been an endlessly patient practical resource, tracking down medical journal articles, tutoring me in some basic principles of immunology, answering questions, and talking over ideas. Once I decided to write the book, Cherry has given unfailing encouragement.

I would like to thank all of the medical professionals who have advised me in the course of my adventure. I have changed their names to protect their privacy, but without exception, they have been knowledgeable, professional, and concerned about my well-being. I also would like to thank the many friends and family who have gone out of their way to accommodate my eating habits.

The final form of this book is due to the work of many talented people at Girl Friday Books, and it has been a pleasure to work with them. I particularly thank Anna Katz, Devon Fredericksen, Ingrid Emerick, Karen Upson, Katie Meyers, Leslie Miller, and Dave Valencia.

In the course of revisions to the book, a number of my friends have read drafts and made observations and suggestions. For that invaluable help, I want to thank Mary Hensley, Tracey Sherry, Ann Robbart, Elayne Aion, Penny McConnell, Clare Holland, and Joan Waltermire. And special thanks to John Douglas for his photograph.

And finally, I say thank you to my beloved Ruth, who applied her sharp editing eye to my work, adapted her culinary gifts to fit my habits, and made every part of my life joyful beyond measure.

SOURCES CONSULTED

Birnbaum, Michael E., Juan L. Mendoza, Dhruv K. Sethi, Shen Dong, Jacob Glanville, Jessica Dobbins, Engin Ozkan, Mark M. Davis, Kai W. Wucherpfennig, and K. Christopher Garcia. "Deconstructing the Peptide-MHC Specificity of T Cell Recognition." *Cell* 157, no. 5 (May 22, 2014): 1073–87. doi: 10.1016/j.cell.2014.03.047.

Boucher, Annie, Marc Desforges, Pierre Duquette, and Pierre J. Talbot. "Long-Term Human Coronavirus-Myelin Cross-Reactive T-Cell Clones Derived from Multiple Sclerosis Patients." *Clinical Immunology* 123, no. 3 (June 2007): 258–67. doi: 10.1016/j.clim.2007.02.002.

Butcher, J. "The Distribution of Multiple Sclerosis in Relation to the Dairy Industry and Milk Consumption." *New Zealand Medical Journal* 83, no. 566 (June 23, 1976): 427–30.

Japan Dairy Council. *Japan Dairy Farming.* Tokyo: Japan Dairy Council, 2011. https://www.dairy.co.jp/jp/engall .pdf.

Malosse, D., H. Perron, A. Sasco, and J. M. Seigneurin. "Correlation between Milk and Dairy Product Consumption and Multiple Sclerosis Prevalence: A Worldwide Study." *Neuroepidemiology* 11, no. 4–6 (1992): 304–12.

Miyake, Sachiko, Sangwan Kim, Wataru Suda, Kenshiro Oshima, Masakazu Nakamura, Takako Matsuoka, Norio Chihara, et al. "Dysbiosis in the Gut Microbiota of Patients with Multiple Sclerosis, with a Striking Depletion of Species Belonging to *Clostridia* XIVa and IV Clusters." *PloS ONE* 10, no. 9 (2015): e0137429. doi: 10.1371/journal.pone.0137429.

Paton, D. J., K. H. Christiansen, S. Alenius, M. P. Cranwell, G. C. Pritchard, and T. W. Drew. "Prevalence of Antibodies to Bovine Virus Diarrhoea Virus and Other Viruses in Bulk Tank Milk in England and Wales." *Veterinary Record* 142, no. 15 (1998): 385–91. doi: 10.1136/vr.142.15.385.

Yamamura, Takashi, and Sachiko Miyake. "Diet, Gut Flora, and Multiple Sclerosis: Current Research and Future Perspectives." In *Multiple Sclerosis Immunology: A Foundation for Current and Future Treatments*, 115–26. New York: Springer, 2012.

ONLINE DATABASES AND ANALYTIC TOOLS

"CTLPred." Elixir bio.tools. Accessed June 5, 2021. https://bio.tools/ctlpred. See also: Bhasin, Manoj, and G. P. S. Raghava, "Prediction of CTL Epitopes Using QM, SVM and ANN Techniques," *Vaccine* 22, no. 23–24 (August 13, 2004): 3195–204, doi: 10.1016/j.vaccine.2004.02.005.

"NETMHCIIpan." DTU Bioinformatics. Updated January 11, 2021. www.cbs.dtu.dk/services/NetMHCIIpan (migrating to DTU Health Tech, updated June 2, 2021, https://services.healthtech.dtu.dk). See also: Reynisson, Birkir, Carolina Barra, Saghar Kaabinejadian, William H. Hildebrand, Bjoern Peters, and Morten Nielsen, "Improved Prediction of MHC II Antigen Presentation through Integration and Motif Deconvolution of Mass Spectrometry MHC Eluted Ligand Data," *Journal of Proteome Research* 19, no. 6 (April 2020): 2304–15, doi: 10.1021/acs.jproteome.9b00874.

"UnitProtKB." UniProt Consortium. Updated February 2, 2021. https://www.uniprot.org/uniprot. See also: UniProt Consortium, "UniProt: A Worldwide Hub of Protein Knowledge," *Nucleic Acids Research* 47, no. D1 (January 8, 2019): D506–15, doi: 10.1093/nar/gky1049.

ABOUT THE AUTHOR

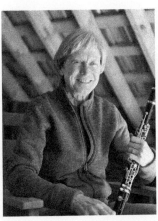

Edith Forbes grew up on a family ranch in Wyoming. She graduated from Stanford University with a degree in English. After a short career in computer programming, she abandoned computers for more earthbound pursuits, including farming and writing. Forbes is the author of the novels *Alma Rose, Nowle's Passing, Exit to Reality,* and *Navigating the Darwin Straits.* Her work is characterized by skillful writing, poignant observations, and quiet yet evocative explorations of the human heart. Recently retired from her farm, she works as a writer and plays as a cross-country skier, gardener, musician, reader, and moviegoer. She lives in Vermont. *Tracking a Shadow* is her first memoir.

CPSIA information can be obtained
at www.ICGtesting.com
Printed in the USA
JSHW040945201221
21386JS00005B/5